FREE

YOURSELF FROM

SMOKING

Dr Kristina Ivings is a practising clinical psychologist whose doctoral thesis explored the relationship between beliefs about smoking and successfully giving up. She has a detailed knowledge of both addictive processes and psychological dependence. She has conducted 'stop smoking' groups and workshops with a remarkable 70% success rate. A former smoker herself, she is passionately committed to helping other people to quit.

FREE

YOURSELF FROM

SMOKING

A 3-point plan to kill
nicotine addiction

KRISTINA IVINGS

Kyle Cathie Ltd

This book is for Edward, Isobel and Katie,
in the hope you never need to read it!

First published in Great Britain in 2006 by
Kyle Cathie Limited
122 Arlington Road
London NW1 7HP
general.enquiries@kyle-cathie.com
www.kylecathie.co.uk

ISBN (10-digit) 1 85626 657 5
ISBN (13-digit) 978 1 85626 657 4

Project editor Caroline Taggart
Copy editor Morag Lyall
Design by www.pinkstripedesign.com
Cartoons by Polyp

Kristina Ivings is hereby identified as the author of this work in accordance with Section 77 of the
Copyright, Designs and Patents Act 1988.

A Cataloguing in Publication record for this title is available from the British Library.

Printed and bound in Great Britain by Cox and Wyman

Contents

Acknowledgements

I would like to thank Margaret Simpson and Sue Khardaji of the Stockport Stop Smoking Service for allowing me to explore my ideas and for supporting me in setting up and running the smoking cessation groups. In addition, I would like to thank Helen Clayton for her valuable contribution to the groups – we always said the one thing missing was a decent book to recommend! And all the smokers who attended my groups, who taught me so much.

Many thanks are due to my friends and family, particularly those who smoke and have found themselves unwittingly featuring in some chapters of this book...

Thank you, too, to Paul Fitzgerald for bringing Nitch to life and to Teresa Chris and Caroline Taggart for making this all possible.

Finally all my gratitude and thanks go to my husband, Mat, for his unfailing love and support – not to mention extra childcare duties!

Preface: who I am & how to use this book

I am a clinical psychologist specialising in smoking. I did my doctorate on smoking and I set up and ran very effective and popular groups for the NHS based on what I discovered in my research.

My approach to helping people stop smoking comes from a branch of psychology called Cognitive Behaviour Therapy (CBT). CBT recognises that people's thoughts, feelings and behaviours are affected by assumptions, beliefs and attitudes that are not necessarily accurate. CBT works by helping people to change the way they think in order to change the way they feel and behave.

As a former smoker, I became fascinated by the psychology of smoking. When I looked at the research evidence and the literature on smoking I discovered that most advice focused on the following things:

- Help to deal directly with the withdrawal symptoms by using patches or other products containing nicotine
- Strategies to help people change their behaviour
- Health education
- Motivational support

What appeared to be missing were ways to help people fundamentally change the way they think about their own smoking and their positive view of cigarettes. The academic literature is full of direct experimental evidence that shows that smoking does not relax people, but rather that smokers are more stressed than non-smokers. It even shows that when people stop smoking their stress levels drop and continue to drop for as long as they remain non-smokers. The psychological literature recognises that smokers are often illogical or irrational and it also stresses the importance of helping smokers change these irrational and inaccurate beliefs if they are going to quit successfully.

But despite these insights, when I spoke to practitioners in the field of smoking they tended to be pessimistic about the chances of changing a belief such as 'Smoking relaxes me'. Even more importantly, some professionals I spoke to did not view statements like 'Smoking relaxes me' or 'I enjoy a cigarette' as merely a belief that might or might not be accurate, but as a statement of fact.

The treatments most commonly offered to smokers do not directly address a crucial part of the smoking trap: distorted positive beliefs about smoking.

In other words, although psychologists had recognised the importance of thoughts, attitudes and beliefs in smoking for a long time, this knowledge was not really being used to help smokers quit.

my research

I therefore decided to research the positive beliefs smokers have about their smoking more fully.

The research questions I was trying to answer were:

• **Do smokers have strong positive beliefs about smoking?**
The answer was yes. (No surprises there!)

• **Can these beliefs be changed?**
The answer to this was also yes. This was exciting confirmation of the fact that smokers really can learn to think and feel differently about their smoking. This was extremely important since many people, including those working in the field of smoking cessation, do not recognise that a lot of what people say

about their own smoking is distorted. Of course, I am not saying that smokers are telling fibs – but they are making mistakes. They do not truly understand their own smoking, so the reasons why they think they smoke are not accurate.

• Does changing their beliefs help people stop smoking?
This time the answer was yes – up to a point. In my research I directly compared therapists (trained by Allen Carr, who kindly co-operated with this research) who focused on changing beliefs with a smoking cessation therapist who focused on behaviour, education, motivation and nicotine replacement products. Both approaches worked about as well as each other. Since people did change their beliefs about smoking, but not all of them stopped smoking, clearly changing beliefs alone is not enough.

I then developed a new approach that combined different aspects of the smoking trap. When I evaluated this combined approach I was excited to see that it was more effective in helping people stop smoking than either approach offered alone.

The approach can be summarised in what I call the Smoking Triangle, which addresses the three factors of physical addiction, psychological dependence and habit. We shall be looking at these in detail in Chapter 2.

Addressing all angles of the Smoking Triangle is much more useful than focusing on just one or two pieces of the puzzle. My approach has been evaluated according to the Department of Health's own strict guidelines and has been proven to be extremely effective. This book therefore gives you the best possible chance of freeing yourself from smoking, permanently!

how to use this book

As we will learn, understanding smoking is more important than willpower when trying to quit. This book explains why most models of smoking are wrong or incomplete. It teaches a new model (the Smoking Triangle), which explains why people smoke and why stopping feels difficult. Once you understand these concepts you can learn to stop more easily, and permanently. Each chapter introduces a new idea or set of ideas that slowly but surely helps you to build up a complete picture of your own smoking.

Most chapters use worksheets which aim to help you learn about, understand and overcome smoking. Please do use the worksheets. I know it might seem a bit like school, but there is plenty of evidence that filling in worksheets really helps. Each chapter finishes with a summary of the key points, which you can return to after you have finished the book to remind you of the main issues.

After we have built up a complete understanding of smoking, and helped you apply it to your own smoking, you come to the main event – how to quit. Please don't turn straight to the 'How to Quit' chapters. You will get there soon enough. You cannot put those chapters into practice until you have built the foundations.

Finally the book teaches you how to stay stopped, and what to do if you are struggling.

Good luck!

Dr Kristina Ivings
June 2005

Why Does Stopping Seem So Difficult?

'It's easy to quit smoking – I've done it a hundred times!'
MARK TWAIN

'Stopping smoking' is a phrase that strikes fear into the hearts of most smokers. The difficulties of quitting are legendary. Almost all smokers have tried to stop, and many have tried dozens and dozens of times. In my Stop Smoking groups a number of people always say despairingly, 'I've tried everything – from acupuncture or hypnotherapy to patches, gums and sprays to sheer willpower or out and out bribery. Nothing works!'

Even those who haven't personally suffered have no doubt heard plenty of horror stories about the difficulties. I hear them myself week after week at the start of the Stop Smoking groups. As people are waiting for everyone to arrive they chat to each other. It makes depressing listening:

- 'A friend of mine whose son is a heroin addict says that stopping smoking is harder than stopping heroin.'
- 'Something like 95% of people fail apparently.'
- 'My wife says she'll leave me if I don't quit but I still don't think I can.'
- 'My doctor says I'll lose the leg unless I stop so now I really have to quit. But then I've been saying that for years.'

We have all heard stories of people continuing to smoke after their legs have been removed, or after heart attacks or surgery for lung cancer. Most of us have met people who quit years ago and still declare that 'not a day goes by when I couldn't murder a cigarette'. This sends a desperately pessimistic message to people who want to stop, making them think, 'If it's really that hard and it never gets any easier, how on earth am I going to do it?'

Other people talk about addiction as an incurable illness. The illness can be controlled but never erased – once a smoker, always a smoker. Yet others view addiction as a character flaw suffered by those with an 'addictive personality'. These widespread beliefs are also shattering to the motivation and self-esteem of a smoker. If it is impossible ever to be truly free of smoking, is it really worth making the effort to quit? The message appears to be crystal clear: Giving up smoking is incredibly difficult. Most people fail. You yourself may have failed on previous attempts. If you try to quit, you have a very good chance of failing again.

No wonder so many smokers choose to ignore their fears about smoking and keep their heads firmly buried in the sand. If they are condemned to lifelong smoking, why torture themselves with all the possible consequences?

Fortunately it does not have to be this way. But it is important to understand the problems if you are going to avoid them. So even if you find the descriptions of quitting depressing, don't be afraid to keep reading!

Why does stopping seem so hard? Why do people feel they cannot stop? To understand the reasons for such high failure rates even among people who are desperate to quit it is necessary to explore the quitting process in detail. Like most things in life there are many ways to go about it. Unfortunately, in the case of smoking, most people choose to go about it the hard way. This is called 'white knuckle quitting' – it even sounds hard.

white knuckle quitting

By far the most common method of quitting is using sheer willpower. If you calculate the costs of smoking and compare them with the benefits, the answer is obvious: the costs far outweigh the benefits, so you should quit. Unfortunately, knowing that smoking is really bad for your health and wallet makes no difference to how much you want a cigarette. In fact the more scared you are of smoking, the more you feel you need to smoke because smoking calms you down!

Think of it as a seesaw. At one end is the desperation to quit and at the other end is the desire to continue. Your mind seesaws back and forth between smoking and stopping. Scared of smoking, but even more scared of life without smoking.

A quit attempt is triggered when the balance tips just far enough towards the stopping smoking end of the seesaw. Perhaps you develop a cough. Perhaps your children ask you to stop. Maybe money is a bit short at the moment or you notice you can no longer walk up the stairs without wheezing. Or perhaps you wake up one Sunday after a night in the pub feeling terrible and think, 'Enough!'

You make the decision to stop and almost immediately doubts and fears creep in. Before their attempt people try to bolster their willpower by marshalling all these excellent reasons firmly in their mind. This is a good way of enhancing motivation – after all there are hundreds of excellent reasons for stopping.

Some people search out pictures of black lungs or write out the stark statistics about smoking to try to scare themselves into stopping. This can work quite well initially. While they are still smoking, the reasons for stopping are in the forefront of their mind. Fear and anxiety about smoking are triggered by each cigarette, thus increasing the desire to stop. Many people manage to stop for a while using this method.

Some people make deals or bargains with themselves or other people. This can feel quite supportive and provide good incentives to keep going with the quit attempt.

These approaches help you to focus on stopping smoking and all can be helpful – up to a point. The problem is none of them makes any difference to how much you want to keep smoking. Wanting to stop doesn't stop you wanting to smoke.

Key Concept

Wanting to stop smoking does not stop you wanting to smoke! No matter how excellent your reasons for stopping are, they don't stop you wanting to smoke the next cigarette.

This is why people think willpower is so important. It feels as if the only way to quit is not to let yourself smoke even though you desperately want to. It seems as though quitting involves gritting your teeth and toughing it out.

So with your long list of reasons to stop smoking, you flex your willpower muscles, firm up your resolve and recite the reasons for quitting to yourself over and over again like a mantra. And then, with a sense of anxiety and loss, you smoke your last cigarette.

Many quit attempts never get beyond the first day. The minute you stub out your last cigarette you want another one. One woman in my group described what happened when she last tried to quit: 'I threw away all my cigarettes, determined that I would do it this time. Ten minutes later I was on my hands and knees fishing them out of the bin again.'

Some people last longer than a day. Some even last a few weeks. At the beginning of a quit attempt the reasons for stopping may be enough to overcome your on-going desire to smoke. But what happens as time goes by?

Well, the obvious change is that you aren't smoking any more. This means your fear and anxiety about smoking are reduced. The pressure has eased and is no longer at the forefront of your mind. But your desire to smoke does not diminish. You want to smoke as much as ever. In fact you often want to smoke more than ever because your memories of smoking take on a rosy glow that bears little resemblance to the reality of smoking. Gradually fear of smoking stops being able to outweigh desire to smoke and your thinking about smoking changes totally. Instead of thinking about the bad aspects of smoking you are now consumed with thoughts of what you are missing out on.

Key Concept

As a quit attempt progresses, fears of smoking fade, while your desire to smoke stays the same or increases. This is why reasons for quitting such as health and cost are seldom enough to stop you smoking permanently.

Once you are in that sort of state of mind you will be looking for a way out. A get-out clause that lets you smoke and makes that decision seem okay to you. And we are all very good at coming up with those…

pick a reason, any reason...

- It's clearly not the right time for me.
- I'm too stressed at the moment.
- Things are too bad at work.
- My family need me to be supportive; they shouldn't be expected to put up with my misery.
- It's selfish of me to continue not smoking when it's affecting me so badly.
- I owe it to my boss to smoke again so I can function properly.
- Just one won't hurt.

The balance tips towards the smoking end of the seesaw and with a sense of relief and release you light up. Ahhhhhhhh that's better! How did you ever imagine life without that wonderful feeling?

why does it go wrong?

When people try white knuckle quitting, the initial motivation to stop can be very powerful. Some admirable people actually do struggle through the misery of the first few days and weeks hoping that one day the cravings will go away. But they don't. In fact they sometimes get worse. No matter how determined that person was to start with, the motivation to keep on with the quit attempt seems to fade while the urge to smoke is as powerful if not more powerful than ever. So why does this happen?

Think of the seesaw again. When a quit attempt was first triggered, all the reasons for stopping were hitting you in the face all day every day. The wheezing, the doctor's lecturing, the expense, the cough, the self-contempt, the children's anxieties, the tensions with your non-smoking spouse, the hassle of going outside to smoke in the rain, the smell, the scary health warnings bombarding you everywhere you turned, the social stigma and so on.

When you stop, those reasons no longer affect you directly. The disadvantages of smoking change from being on-going stressful experiences to mere *memories*. And memories simply do not have the impact of real experiences. So the motivation for quitting begins to slide a little bit as the misery of smoking fades into memory.

But what about the advantages of the smoking end of the seesaw? That hasn't changed! In fact the pleasures and benefits of smoking get elevated higher than when you were actually smoking. Recent ex-smokers put smoking high on a pedestal. They remember all the 'best' cigarettes and think wistfully of all those wonderful smokes in lovely places, erasing the thousands of forgettable cigarettes or the uncomfortable cigarettes in inconvenient places.

People start making random associations between cigarettes and good times. If they see a smiling smoker they think, 'That guy is smiling *because he is smoking*!' So while the costs are fading the benefits are becoming hugely exaggerated, with the result that the seesaw tips back towards smoking and the quit attempt fails.

Key Concept

People who quit smoking put cigarettes on a pedestal. They then crave something that is better than the real thing!

Whatever your smoking history and whatever the costs of smoking are to you, the balance almost always tips back towards smoking in the end. Older smokers often think younger smokers could stop easily because they are not so severely addicted. On the other hand, younger smokers firmly believe that they would never let themselves get to the stage of ill health and disability before quitting. The truth is that all smokers are caught in a similar trap. Whether you are younger or older, smoke two a day or eighty a day, you are all stuck in the Smoking Triangle (see Chapter 2) and will all experience similar problems in quitting.

The basic problem is that for some reason the misery of quitting seems directly proportional to the misery of smoking and so you stay in the trap. If you decide to quit because you tell yourself that you'd quite like to stop smoking, you can let yourself off the hook by telling yourself you'd quite like to start again now. Whereas if you tell yourself you absolutely have to stop because it is killing you, you also feel that you can't live without it. The more desperate you are to stop, the more desperate you are to continue. So no matter how bad smoking gets, the fear of stopping is as great or greater than the fear of continuing. People sense that they are stuck, and that they can't escape. It feels like the ultimate Catch-22. But don't panic! This book will explain why that happens, and show you how to overcome the problem.

Key Concept

Your desperation to stop is balanced by your desire to continue. So the more you want to stop, the harder stopping feels.

It is important to recognise that our thoughts actually change when we start to smoke again. Thoughts such as:

- 'I'm scared of getting ill' suddenly change to 'We all die some time'.
- 'I want to get fitter' becomes 'I can take up sport even if I smoke – balance is the key'.
- 'Smoking is a horrible habit' changes to 'Smoking is intensely pleasurable'.
- 'I'm sick of being a slave to a drug' becomes 'Cigarettes are always there for me, they never let me down'.
- 'It's embarrassing and anti-social when I have to go outside and smoke' is now seen as 'Social situations are difficult without smoking' or 'Smokers are more interesting people'.
- 'I don't want to die young' shifts to 'I'd rather die young and happy than be a grumpy, miserable old git!'

Once your own mind has started rebelling against your self-imposed cigarette deprivation you are on your way to smoking again.

As you may well know from your own experiences, once you are back on the slippery slope your attempt to quit is doomed. One or two on a Saturday night becomes eight or ten on Friday and Saturday nights. Then you start smoking whenever you are in a pub so Wednesdays become smoking days too. Then you start going to the pub more than ever before to give yourself an excuse to smoke! Then you start buying them again because your friends have got sick of you scrounging all the time. Before you know it you are back on forty a day and feeling more depressed and hopeless than ever.

fear of smoking versus fear of stopping...

One of the problems with quitting is that smokers feel that there are basically only two options. And neither is attractive. First, you can stay as you are and keep on smoking. This is, of course, an expensive and unhealthy option but you won't be any worse off than you are now.

Smokers are good at hiding things from themselves. They are masters at the art of sticking their head in the sand and ignoring the grim realities of living (and dying) a smoker. Many smokers smoke for years on end and the thought of quitting never enters their heads. They simply feel that the misery of stopping would be unbearable, so they dismiss that option. They then have to try as hard as possible to ignore the misery of continuing and just try to make a virtue out of the necessity of keeping on puffing.

These are the 'die-hard' smokers who almost make a career out of their smoking. They believe that smokers are more interesting, that the best conversations at parties are outside where all the smokers are, that quitting is for holier-than-thou prigs or health freaks and that smoking truly and deeply enhances their lives. They often wear their ill health (such as a gravelly voice) like a badge of honour. They learn to blow elaborate smoke rings, do tricks with Zippos or buy gold lighters. They tell jokes like 'I never get sick – no germs could survive in my body.'

Much as they might protest to the contrary, these people are just as keen to stop as every other smoker, and if a magic pill came onto the market that cured nicotine addiction immediately they would jump at it. In fact they do jump at it. Every so often a 'cure' for smoking is launched. It happened recently with Zyban. It is the confirmed smokers who are first in line for those sorts of treatments. These smokers' basic problem is that while they long to be free as much as everyone else, they believe it is impossible without some 'magic' to take away their desire to smoke.

The second option is quitting. For those who do summon up the courage to try, the quitting option leads to real fear as the person imagines a future of endless deprivation and misery. Never enjoying a cup of coffee, or a meal, or an evening in the pub again. Never having the ability to reduce stress. Never being able to cope. As John Reid, then UK Secretary of State for Health, remarked in early 2004, some people even feel that smoking is one of their few pleasures! With such strong beliefs about the attractions of smoking it is no wonder that quitting seems a pretty unattractive option too, but at least you would save money and make significant health and fitness gains.

Unfortunately, anyone who tries to quit is likely to enter the attempt with the real fear that they might fail. This fear is a powerful barrier to any serious attempt to stop. Even friends and family grow weary of the oft-heard phrase 'I'm giving up smoking' and respond with scepticism if not outright derision. If no one else believes you can do it, it doesn't do much for your own confidence. Being a smoker is bad enough at the best of times, but when people are smoking freely without thinking about quitting, they often manage to keep their head in the sand and ignore some of the risks and costs associated with it. A quit attempt involves taking their head out of the sand and admitting that they *hate* being a smoker, that they are *terrified* of the implications of smoking and they are *utterly* sick and tired of needing to smoke no matter how inconvenient.

Taking a long, hard, honest look at your smoking and the effect it has on your life is fine if you then go on to quit. But what if you can't? What if you make these frightening admissions about how much you hate smoking, only to end up smoking again anyway?

don't despair!

Now that I have thoroughly depressed you, I can assure you that it doesn't have to be this way. There is another way – to quit and be delighted to be shot of cigarettes, to feel free and never to miss them at all. This may sound like an impossible dream, but it is possible and is already a wonderful reality for many ex-smokers.

This book will show you how to:

- Quit without misery and fear.
- Never miss cigarettes.
- Take cravings in your stride.
- Feel totally confident in your ability to succeed.
- Experience less stress and misery.
- Quit with a feeling of relief and freedom rather than anxiety or dread.

Despite the fact that many people find it hard to stay stopped, many others do succeed permanently and live perfectly happily without wanting or missing cigarettes. Many of you may have experienced this happy state in the past.

Often people who have failed in a quit attempt are doubly disappointed because they actually didn't find it that hard to stop. But for some weird reason, even though they stopped before and it was quite easy, they can't do so again now. Or people who just decide to stop and do so with few problems are pleasantly surprised but a bit puzzled at their success.

In my groups at least half the people say they have stopped for months or even years in the past and had no problems with stopping. But they started again for one reason or another and now have no idea how they ever managed without cigarettes. Even these people view being happy as a non-smoker as an impossible dream – although they themselves have been happy as non-smokers in the past. This is a good example of how the addiction affects thinking and reasoning. When you are addicted, being free of the addiction seems impossible. Yet as soon as you are free, you can't imagine ever getting hooked again.

In fact we have all been happy to be non-smokers in the past – before we started smoking. Wouldn't it be nice if you could get back to the happy innocence of not being remotely bothered by cigarettes? Well, you can. That is precisely what you can achieve with this book.

Key Concept

No matter what your smoking history, you can be completely free of smoking.

It is perfectly possible to be permanently and totally free, no matter how badly you are addicted at the moment. But it is virtually impossible to control smoking, no matter how easy it was to quit. In practical terms this means:

- Yes, you can quit!
- No, you can't have the odd one now and again!

Where so many smokers go wrong is that they believe the opposite statements to be true. When they are smoking they tell themselves they can't stop (not true!). But when they have stopped they tell themselves they are safe to smoke occasionally without getting hooked again (also not true).

The lucky people who stop without feeling miserable have stumbled accidentally on a frame of mind that allows them to quit.

But they don't understand how they got there. They don't know why they have succeeded in stopping smoking this time. So if they get caught by smoking again, they don't have the knowledge they need to escape.

Don't worry if you are not one of those people who have stopped without too much difficulty in the past. In my groups many people say that they have stopped before but found it a horrible miserable experience which was much too hard to sustain. These people can also stop easily and permanently. Others have never stopped for even a day before. They can also quit. So whatever your smoking and quitting history, you too can succeed in your dream of being totally free of all desire to smoke.

The aim of this book is to teach you the secrets of successful quitting. The key to successful and permanent quitting is to understand smoking.

Key Concept

> **Smokers do not need to be superhuman to quit! Understanding smoking is more important than willpower.**

chapter summary

• Everyone 'knows' how hard it is to quit. They are wrong.

• Most people quit using sheer willpower, or 'white knuckle quitting'.

• This is indeed very hard...

• Understanding smoking is more important than willpower.

Worksheet

Getting started!
The first step to the new smoke-free you is to understand your own smoking. Fill in this table with everything good and everything bad about cigarettes that you can think of.

+	−

Why Do People Smoke?

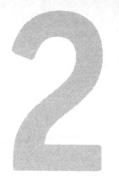

Smoking is full of paradoxes and contradictions. Until you can understand the following things, you will not be truly free:

- Nicotine addiction is vague, subtle and often barely noticeable and nicotine addiction is a tremendously powerful force.
- You don't enjoy smoking and smoking feels extremely enjoyable at times.
- Smoking reduces your anxiety and smoking makes you anxious.
- Nicotine withdrawal only takes a few days and cravings to smoke can hit you months or years after stopping.
- You can get hooked on something you loathe doing.

Most importantly, you need to understand all aspects of the smoking problem. You need to know how your mind works against you in order to keep you smoking, or to make you start again if you have stopped. And you need to understand why the drive to smoke *does not respond to logical reasoning* – which is why you cannot talk yourself out of wanting to smoke.

In most quit attempts people think about all the reasons for stopping and don't pay too much attention to reasons for carrying on. After all, the pleasures and benefits of smoking are obvious… Aren't they?

Actually, no. The question of why people smoke in the face of appalling costs is not immediately obvious. Yes, it's an addiction, but that is a description, not an explanation. Most people do not truly understand their own reasons for smoking and are not very good at explaining smoking – despite the fact that most people think they are!

Various psychological theories have been put forward over the years to try to explain smoking. But they don't answer the question very well either.

An example is the 'three-stage model'[1] which claims that people smoke as a result of the interaction between three factors. The first is called 'psychosocial reinforcement' which covers things like peer pressure or the desire to be sociable. For example, smoking at a party when someone offers you a cigarette in order to break the ice, or to be friendly.

The second factor is 'positive reinforcement' and refers to getting pleasures or benefits from smoking, such as improved mood, better concentration or relaxation.

The final factor is 'negative reinforcement', which means doing something in order to avoid or remove something unpleasant. For example, smoking removes withdrawal symptoms.

In other words, this model suggests that people smoke because other people they know are doing it, because they get pleasures and benefits from it and because if they don't do it unpleasant things happen. Sounds reasonable? Perhaps it seems to make sense because this is a description of virtually any behaviour – going for a jog, eating a chocolate bar, having sex, going to work. Most rational behaviours are influenced by what that behaviour can help you get – and by what it can help you avoid.

There is an inaccurate assumption among health professionals and smokers themselves that whether or not a person smokes is governed by the same sort of rational decision-making as any other behaviour. This view suggests that smokers weigh up the pros and cons and make a choice about whether or not to smoke. The researcher who developed the three-stage model wrote: 'Decisions are based ultimately on the subjectively perceived balance of advantages and disadvantages of smoking...the decision is always a rational one from the subject's viewpoint.'[2]

This sort of theory is not good at explaining addictions. (And if you are a smoker, I can assure you that are addicted to nicotine.) The assumption that smoking feels rational, even to smokers themselves, simply does not tie in with the actual experience of being in an addiction trap. One heroin addict wrote:

> Hunting for a reason to stop that outweighs the drive to stay hooked is the major problem. During one soul-searching session I neatly listed advantages and disadvantages of taking smack. Potential consequences of using heroin included being charged with an offence, starring in a scandal, losing home, job, wealth, friends and credibility of every kind. Advantages were impossible to find. The following statements appeared on the list of reasons not to stop: 'It [heroin] makes life easier'; 'I'm scared to stop' and 'I don't feel like it'. A moment's thought contradicted the first two and left me confronted by the third. I did not 'feel like it'. I did not stop.[3]

Cigarettes are not heroin, and smokers are not heroin addicts, but cigarettes and heroin are both highly addictive. While there are many differences between smoking and illegal drug use, the addictive processes behind all drug use are the same. As this passage highlights, no matter what they are addicted to, the addiction makes people behave in ways that are not rational – *and they know it.*

The actual experience of addiction is effectively captured by C. S. Lewis, who wrote of 'an ever-increasing craving for an ever-diminishing pleasure'. [4] This is a much better description of how it feels to be desperate to smoke cigarettes that you don't even really enjoy.

Smokers are addicts. And they behave in ways that are not rational. This means that rational 'reasons' for smoking may not be the real reasons that people smoke. Addiction and addictive processes are covered in detail in Chapter 4.

the smoking triangle

This book describes a different model of smoking from the 'three stages' mentioned above. I call it the Smoking Triangle. It is explained fully later on, but in summary it represents three separate problems that smokers have to overcome in order to free themselves from smoking.

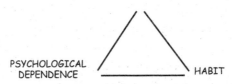

PHYSICAL ADDICTION

PSYCHOLOGICAL DEPENDENCE

HABIT

• Physical addiction: cigarettes are addictive, so part of the problem is that you need nicotine in order to feel okay. You feel anxious or edgy without it.

• Psychological dependence: you have strong positive beliefs about smoking that make the prospect of quitting seem scary and miserable.

- Habit: you tend to smoke in the same places and at the same times, and those situations feel weird and difficult if you don't smoke.

Key Concept

> **Smokers are nicotine addicts. Addicted thinking is not rational thinking.**

so what reasons do people give for why they smoke?

Why do people smoke? On the face of it, it seems a bizarre thing to do. Research has shown that 90% of smokers want to quit.[5] Smoking is widely recognised as Britain's biggest preventable killer – killing 120,000 people every year. Everywhere you go you are bombarded with anti-smoking information. Society is becoming more and more intolerant of smokers. Office workers are forced to go outside to smoke no matter what the weather. Every Budget Day smokers wince again as the cost of smoking goes up and up. At the moment the cost to a family that smokes forty a day between them is roughly equivalent to that of a £60,000 mortgage!

These costs have not stopped you smoking. Being scared of the consequences is not enough to stop you doing it. Ironically, the more scared you are, the more you feel you need a cigarette! The problem is that you are smoking for a reason. After all, you aren't stupid or mad. If you are putting up with all this in order to smoke, you must be getting something in return. Cigarettes seem to be able to do things for you that you can't get from anything else. Everyone has their own reasons for smoking, but most fall into the following categories:

relaxation and stress reduction

Smoking is relaxing and relieves stress. Smoking helps you cope with life's difficulties. Smoking gives you courage and confidence to tackle difficult situations. In times of stress cigarettes are always there for you – endlessly reliable, ever dependable.

Imagine taking an exam or driving test. The cigarette does its magic before the test to help you cope with your nerves. After the test the cigarette is there again ready to help you unwind. Or imagine being stuck on a delayed flight stacked above Heathrow for hours waiting to land. Finally your plane is diverted to Geneva where you face a night on a bench in the airport. There's little information and no compensation. You are cold, tired, frustrated and angry. You finally get outside where you can light up. Take a deep drag right down to your toes and feel the stress ebbing away instantly. Can you imagine coping without it?

concentration

Smoking sharpens you up. Smoking helps you to focus. Smoking gets your brain in gear. Think of the cliché of the overworked writer – fag in one hand, bottle of Jack Daniels in the other. When I was a smoker and I had a problem at work, a cigarette always seemed to help me sort it out. I could have a smoke and think the problem through. The smoke somehow made me think more clearly so I would find a solution. Smoking gives you that extra edge of creativity. Think of having to make a difficult phone call. A cigarette in hand gives you extra confidence to succeed. On long car journeys, cigarettes can keep you alert and focused. You have to make an important presentation and are up late working on it – cigarettes help you to stay sharp. How could you cope with the demands of a stressful life without cigarettes to give you a helping hand?

enjoyment

'A woman is only a woman but a good cigar is a Smoke,' said Rudyard Kipling. Smoking is immeasurably pleasurable, gratifyingly satisfying. The taste, smell, sensation of inhaling and even the way the smoke curls seductively up into the air are all deeply satisfying pleasures. Merely the sight of a shiny new packet can lift your spirits. Unwrapping the cellophane, extracting the cigarette, the sharp flare of the match or the satisfying click of the Zippo. All aspects of smoking are enjoyable.

making good times better

No activities are complete without a smoke to go with them. No meal out would give pleasure if you couldn't smoke afterwards. A coffee without a ciggy is like strawberries without cream. Can you imagine beers or cocktails on a lovely holiday evening without a cigarette to go with them? Life without smoking would be duller and drearier.

addiction

Quitting creates terrible withdrawal symptoms. If you stop you'll climb the walls with cravings. You will be tense, irritable and thoroughly miserable. Your misery affects everyone around you, making them pray that you'll start smoking again because you are so unbearable to live with. Would your relationships even survive a quit attempt? And anyway once an addict always an addict. You might quit for years and years but never a day will go by when you won't feel that you could murder a cigarette. Is it really worth all this misery?

So smoking makes good times better, bad times less bad, improves your concentration, is deeply enjoyable and satisfying, helps relax you and helps you cope with the stresses and strains of life. No wonder you don't want to give all that up.

At this point you may be suspecting that I am actually a Philip Morris plant! I appear to be trying to persuade you how fantastic smoking is. If smoking really does all the above and more, then no wonder you smoke. And no wonder you are scared of stopping. If this were all true, the puzzle would be not that so many people smoke, but that anyone ever manages to give it up at all.

However, the truth, as you may be suspecting, is not so simple… Frankly, if cigarettes did all that for me, I'd still be smoking too. However, even though you might guess (quite rightly) that there is more to these 'benefits' than meets the eye, it is very, very important that you fully understand what you think you get from a cigarette before you try to quit.

Key Concept

The reasons you think you smoke may not be the real reasons you smoke.

- 'Reasons' for smoking make you too scared even to try to stop.
- 'Reasons' for smoking make success less likely if you do summon enough courage to try.
- 'Reasons' for smoking make your quit attempt feel miserable.
- 'Reasons' for smoking make it more likely that you will eventually go back to smoking if you do stop.

What a tragedy it would be if these 'reasons' were in fact false and flawed when they are so important in condemning you to lifelong smoking. You owe it to yourself to explore them.

chapter summary

- 'Commonsense' models of smoking are wrong.

- Smokers have many reasons for smoking.

- These reasons make stopping seem difficult.

- Understanding your own reasons for smoking is essential if you are to be truly free.

Worksheet

TICK ALL THE STATEMENTS THAT YOU AGREE WITH IN THE FOLLOWING QUESTIONNAIRE.[6]

1 Cigarettes taste nice.

2 Not smoking is uncomfortable.

3 Smokers put cigarettes in their mouths without noticing.

4 Being without cigarettes is very unpleasant.

5 Cigarettes ease social situations.

6 Cigarettes help people forget their worries.

7 Cigarettes prevent people slowing down.

8 Cigarettes make people look sophisticated or grown up.

9 Handling cigarettes is part of the enjoyment of smoking.

10 Some people smoke for taste alone.

11 Being without cigarettes is almost unbearable.

12 People smoke automatically without being aware of it.

13 Smoking helps at parties if you don't know anyone there.

14 Smoking helps ease embarrassment.

15 It looks good to be smoking.

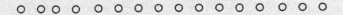

16 Smoking is sociable.

17 Smoking gives you something to do with your mouth.

18 Smoking helps people be more at ease with other people.

19 Smoking can keep people awake.

20 Flicking ash is one of the pleasures of smoking.

21 Smoking cigarettes is pleasant and relaxing.

22 Stopping smoking creates a really gnawing hunger.

23 Smoking is stimulating and perks people up.

24 Smoking helps people be one of the crowd.

25 Part of the enjoyment of smoking comes from the steps you need to take to light up.

26 Cigarettes are pleasurable.

27 Life is easier if you can smoke.

Now have another look at the seesaw you did for the first worksheet.

Using the seesaw, the reasons described in this chapter, and the questionnaire, write a long list of everything you get from smoking. Ignore reasons for quitting at the moment. Instead concentrate on the things you like about cigarettes or the things you get from them.

○ ○ ○ ○ ○ ○ ○ ○ ○ ○ ○ ○ ○ ○ ○ ○

Worksheet cont'd

Make this list as long as possible and write it in as much detail as possible. This is very important because even though you want to quit, you also want to carry on. It is the reasons for wanting to carry on that make a quit attempt fail. So you need to be really clear about what you think about cigarettes.

Do not read further until you have finished this work sheet! It won't take long!

A New Understanding of Smoking: meet Nitch

Now that I have just about convinced you that smoking is a great and wonderful thing to do despite its unfortunate costly side effects I am going to state categorically that all the above is not true. Smoking does not give you any of the benefits or pleasures I have just described. In fact smoking does not achieve anything worthwhile for you at all.

I know this sounds a bit much to accept – after all, you *actually experience* the pleasures and benefits that I am claiming do not exist. So on the one hand I am agreeing that you may indeed experience cigarettes as relaxing, confidence-enhancing, concentration-boosting, stress-relieving and enjoyable, but also that these pleasures and benefits don't exist.

In other words: you smoke. You enjoy it. It makes you feel better. But smoking is neither enjoyable nor helpful.

Huh?

Be patient, it will all become clear. One secret of successful quitting is to sort out this apparent paradox – to understand how cigarettes trap you into believing they help you when in fact all the benefits are costs in disguise.

Key Concept

'Benefits' of smoking are really costs in disguise.

To understand how thoroughly you can be fooled into believing the myths about cigarettes you need to meet a little creature called Nitch. Nitch stands for Nicotine Itch, and Itch stands for:

- Irritating
- Time consuming
- Controlling
- Horrible

introducing Nitch

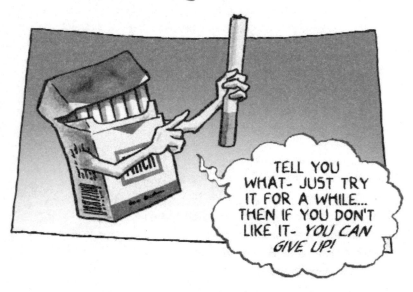

TELL YOU WHAT- JUST TRY IT FOR A WHILE... THEN IF YOU DON'T LIKE IT- *YOU CAN GIVE UP!*

Meet Nitch. He's a little parasite who lives inside you. He feeds on nicotine. When he has nicotine he is as quiet as a little mouse. When he is deprived of nicotine he winds you up and stresses you out. In terms of not taking no for an answer, Nitch is in a league of his own. Nitch needs nicotine to live. Without a regular supply he will

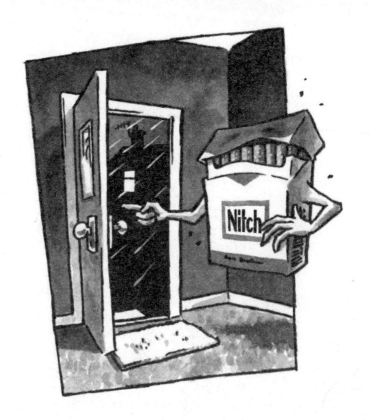

die. He depends on you to keep him supplied. He needs to make certain that his supplier (i.e. *you*) continues to feed him no matter how expensive or inconvenient that may be, and no matter what the health cost to you.

Nitch doesn't care if the nearest cigarettes are in the twenty-four-hour garage ten miles away and it's blowing a blizzard outside. It's nothing to *him* if getting cigarettes means not being able to afford food. So how does he manage to make assertive and independent people quite such slaves to his desires?

Everyone who smokes has Nitch inside them. You too have a Nitch that lives in you. Nitch has two weapons: **anxiety** and **propaganda**.

anxiety

When people smoke, the following cycle occurs over and over again.

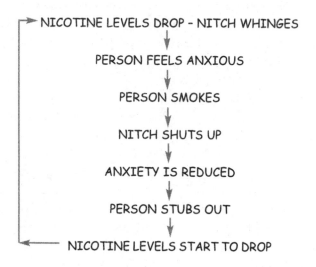

NICOTINE LEVELS DROP - NITCH WHINGES
↓
PERSON FEELS ANXIOUS
↓
PERSON SMOKES
↓
NITCH SHUTS UP
↓
ANXIETY IS REDUCED
↓
PERSON STUBS OUT
↓
NICOTINE LEVELS START TO DROP

Nitch makes a fuss as soon as the nicotine levels in your blood drop. He makes himself a nuisance by making you feel tense or anxious. When you smoke, the feeling vanishes instantly. So the cigarette is experienced as relaxing and relieving. But by smoking you guarantee that the tension and anxiety return as soon as Nitch feels hungry again.

This feeling of anxiety is caused by nicotine withdrawal. In other words it is an artificial, chemically induced anxiety. But it feels no less real for that. We are all powerfully motivated to reduce anxiety, because anxiety is a danger signal. Our unconscious mind thinks that when we experience anxiety it is because there is some danger around, and it prompts us to do whatever it takes to reduce the anxiety. This strong unconscious drive to reduce anxiety is nothing to do with how unpleasant anxiety itself is – early flickerings of anxiety are not painful. The strong drive to reduce anxiety is actually a survival mechanism because our unconscious mind thinks that **anxiety = danger** and it wants us to get away from the danger.

Usually this mechanism works just fine. If we stand too near a cliff edge we feel a little anxious, so we move back a few steps. This is helpful behaviour. It goes wrong when the anxiety is caused not by danger but by the chemical reactions triggered in nicotine withdrawal. In this case, the drive to reduce the anxiety by whatever it takes leads us to make a mistake. We learn very quickly that smoking reduces this anxiety. So we smoke. This is not a rational attempt to make ourselves feel better, but a biologically driven attempt to reduce anxiety (and therefore make us more likely to survive).

After we stub out a cigarette Nitch is only quiet for a few minutes. Then slowly but surely he starts whining again. Smokers are so used to this that they barely know Nitch is there. He has them so well trained that he just has to give a little peep and they obligingly light up again, sometimes without even noticing they are doing it.

In my groups some smokers always say that they don't know why they smoke most of the cigarettes they smoke as they 'get nothing from them'. In fact they do get something from them – a bit more peace from Nitch. It's just that if they respond to Nitch quickly, before he gets into a real strop, they barely notice the difference when they shut him up.

In psychological terms this process is called **negative reinforcement**. A reinforcer is something that increases the likelihood of a behaviour being repeated. **Positive reinforcement** means increasing the likelihood of the behaviour by giving something desirable when the behaviour occurs. For example, eating chocolate is positively reinforced because it tastes delicious. Negative reinforcement means increasing the likelihood of a behaviour because the behaviour removes something undesirable, such as anxiety.

Anything we do that reduces anxiety is reinforced, so we are more likely to do it again. In smoking, the anxiety is chemically induced. There is no real danger. But the survival mechanism is not sophisticated enough to tell the difference between anxiety born of real danger and anxiety created by nicotine withdrawal.

This is the first angle in the Smoking Triangle: the physical drive to smoke, arising from physical addiction.

Key Concept

We are *programmed* to reduce anxiety by whatever means possible. This is a biological survival mechanism.

Let's think again about Nitch. Whenever he makes a fuss and you feed him you are rewarded. So your smoking behaviour is reinforced – over and over again, hundreds of times a week. If you try to limit your smoking Nitch gets more and more upset with you and makes more and more of a fuss. When you do finally give in, you reduce more anxiety and the relief feels tremendous. This is why some cigarettes are experienced as amazingly wonderful while others aren't that big a deal. When we are smoking freely we barely notice the anxiety. But when we limit smoking there is a greater amount of anxiety when we do finally smoke, so the cigarette is experienced as more satisfying.

The most 'enjoyable' cigarettes are the ones after a period without smoking, for example, first thing in the morning, straight after getting off a flight, after a meal or when we get in from work. These cigarettes are simply the ones that end a bigger Nitch tantrum. The illusion is that they are 'better' than the ones we chain-smoke in a pub. But the reality is that Nitch made us more anxious before the 'best' cigarettes, so we experienced greater relief when we shut him up. This is exactly the same process that makes food taste so much better when we are hungry – the hungrier we are, the more rewarding eating is.

The anxiety caused by Nitch builds up gradually over time. It is also vague, subtle and no different from the general anxieties of life. So smokers don't recognise that Nitch is making them anxious. Their impression is that they feel a bit better whenever they smoke. In fact the situation is that smokers are almost permanently stressed by Nitch and what feels 'better' is simply the temporary removal of this chemically induced state of anxiety.

It has been known for a long time that smokers are more stressed than non-smokers. People used to believe that this was because people who had more stressful lives tended to smoke. In fact research has now shown that even if you take all other factors into account, smokers are still more stressed and unhappy than non-smokers.[7] When people stop smoking their stress levels begin to drop and they carry on dropping for as long as they stay off the cigarettes.[8] People who start smoking again only show rises in stress levels *after* starting again, which proves that they do not simply start smoking again because they are stressed.

In addition, smokers are much more likely to develop stress-related disorders such as agoraphobia, panic disorder and generalised anxiety disorder than non-smokers.

So it is quite clear that far from helping you deal with stress, cigarettes actually *cause* anxiety. And no wonder! Having Nitch living in you, giving you hassle whenever he gets a little low on nicotine, is incredibly stressful. It's like carrying around a permanent parasite you can never get rid of even for a few hours. Nitch will never learn any manners or patience and will never go away. He doesn't understand the words 'no' or 'later'. He is as persistently irritating as a toddler in the chocolate aisle of a supermarket. And he gradually gets stronger and stronger as his need for nicotine increases.

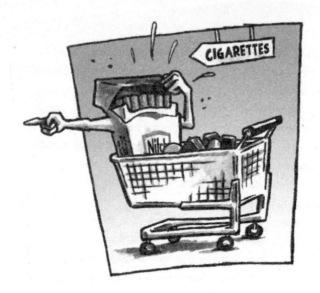

Smoking is no more than an attempt to be free of Nitch's whining. Smokers spend their lives trying to rid themselves of the aggravation of this little pest. But by smoking they are merely keeping him alive and well, ready to irritate and distract them some more in a little while.

Key Concept

> **Nitch causes anxiety. Smoking appears to be helpful because smoking shuts Nitch up for a while. But it also keeps him alive, so that he can stress you out again.**

So how does he get away with it? Basically, Nitch's power is in the timing of the anxiety. When they think of smoking, most people think about what is happening while they are actually smoking.

But you are a smoker twenty-four hours a day, so it is just as legitimate to look at a different part of the cycle. Let's start with stubbing out. After you stub out a cigarette you enter a period of nicotine withdrawal, which causes anxiety. When you smoke, Nitch shuts up and the anxiety vanishes. This relief is almost instant, and it is perfectly obvious that it is the cigarette that has made you feel better.

However, the feeling of wanting to smoke is an entirely artificial feeling that was created when you got hooked on smoking. The stress of needing to smoke is caused by nothing other than smoking. This smoking-related anxiety builds up gradually, and so the smoker does not link it with nicotine withdrawal and the last cigarette they had. So cigarettes get all the credit for calming you down but none of the blame for stressing you out.

Key Concept

Cigarettes get all the credit for calming you down, but none of the blame for stressing you out in the first place.

The feeling of wanting to smoke is an entirely artificial feeling that was created when you started smoking.

People view smoking as a welcome pleasure in a stressful world. So giving up is seen as the loss of something truly precious. The reality however is that Nitch is an unwanted intruder in your life that creates anxiety and never leaves you alone. Quitting simply means freeing yourself from the misery of life with Nitch.

Nitch's ability to stress you out is, however, only one weapon in his armoury. Even more powerful is his phenomenally successful use of propaganda.

propaganda

People will believe virtually anything positive about smoking. They will also disbelieve virtually anything negative. How and why this total bias in our thinking arises is crucial in understanding the secrets of successful quitting.

We humans greatly dislike a psychological state called **cognitive dissonance**. Cognitive means to do with the mind or thoughts. Dissonance means conflict. So cognitive dissonance refers to a state of mind in which a person has conflicting thoughts about something. A clear example of this would be the two thoughts 'Smoking causes cancer' and 'I smoke'. Cognitive dissonance often arises when people are secretly unhappy about the way they have behaved or are behaving.

The same process can be seen in many areas of life. People like to be able to justify their behaviour. We don't much care if we are right, as long as we believe we are right!

Smoking creates massive amounts of cognitive dissonance because people are repeatedly doing something that they know is deadly. Smokers are in the terrible position of continuing to carry out a behaviour that scares them, destroys their health and costs them lots of money.

To add to their miseries is the fact that they seem to get so little in return for these devastating financial and physical costs. I mean *why* do people smoke? There is little physical or emotional change. Smokers do not experience euphoric effects. Nicotine is not an intoxicant. There is no high associated with smoking. The 'buzz' or 'head rush' very young or inexperienced smokers describe simply reflects an intolerance to nicotine which vanishes when they become addicted.

When you first start to smoke you experience smoking as revolting and horrible – and the cigarettes don't change. They taste as horrible after ten years as they did at first. If you have 'developed a taste' for them, this is just another example of changing beliefs instead of behaviour. Don't believe me? Have you actually tasted one recently?! Light one now – go on, I'll wait. In fact you'd better smoke two. The first one will get rid of Nitch, who disguises the taste.

Ready with the second cigarette? Ten deep drags and focus on the taste and sensation. Mmmmm?

Since smoking has such enormous costs and offers remarkably little in return, smokers find themselves in the very uncomfortable position of behaving in a way they don't like. They need to relieve this discomfort and they do this by developing strong and powerful beliefs about the benefits and pleasures of smoking.

This is where Nitch's propaganda machine comes in. You need a justification to smoke. And Nitch is only too happy to provide you with hundreds of them.

Remember the benefits and pleasures of smoking we talked about earlier? Well, that is Nitch at his best. He manages to make you believe that cigarettes calm you down, sharpen you up, help you focus, help you unwind, aid your concentration, keep you alert, help you sleep, enhance your enjoyment of any activity, ease the pain of any misfortune and provide pleasure and satisfaction.

Smokers come to believe that, okay, they aren't happy about the health stuff, but, hey, smoking does so much for them! If they didn't smoke they couldn't work, enjoy themselves or relax. They would be grumpy and miserable all the time for ever and ever. Faced with a choice of quitting and being irritable and miserable or keeping on smoking, people usually choose smoking. But the secret of successful stopping is that *you don't have to feel miserable and deprived if you stop!*

It cannot be emphasised enough that the benefits are costs in disguise. And it is so easy to be fooled because they are widely regarded, not just by smokers but by non-smokers and even by health professionals, as genuine effects of smoking.

The questionnaire that you filled in on page 36 was adapted from a widely accepted and much-used questionnaire developed by a respected scientist called Tomkins in 1966. Turn back and look at it again. The scientist who came up with all those reasons for smoking believed that they were genuine effects of smoking. If a top scientist in the field was fooled by all this, no wonder you believe it too. The secret of successful quitting is to understand that these are not reasons for smoking, but *justifications for smoking to make you feel better about it!*

Key Concept

'Reasons' for smoking are really justifications to make you feel better about it.

The tragedy about developing these inaccurate beliefs is that they then present a formidable barrier to quitting. A person isn't just giving up an anti-social, unhealthy and expensive behaviour, but a highly valued, stress-relieving, confidence-enhancing, ever-reliable friend.

The joy of quitting is the recognition that all these perceived benefits are false promises and that when you stop you find yourself wallowing happily in the benefits that you thought cigarettes gave you.

In a study I carried out in 1998 I gave people the Reasons for Smoking Questionnaire before and after treatment that aimed to change their positive view of smoking. The good news is that the research showed that these beliefs can easily be altered.

summary of Nitch's dastardly deeds

The feelings of anxiety that Nitch creates when he wants feeding are withdrawal symptoms. Withdrawal is not something you go through when you are quitting. Withdrawal is what you are going through all day every day and will continue to go through all day every day for as long as you continue to smoke.

Smoking is a hopelessly doomed attempt to get rid of Nitch. He stresses you out and makes you anxious. So you smoke to make him go away. But by smoking you keep him alive, ready and willing to come back to stress you out and make you anxious again.

You are driven to smoke by a basic misunderstanding. Your unconscious mind thinks that anxiety = danger and you are motivated to do whatever it takes to reduce anxiety. So you smoke. But the danger signals are faulty. The misunderstanding has conned you into smoking, which makes you feel uncomfortable because you know as well as anyone how devastating smoking is to your health. Nitch doesn't want you to be too worried about these things in case they persuade you to stop his supply of nicotine. He therefore convinces you that the fears are exaggerated or somehow don't apply to you, while at the same time putting cigarettes on a pedestal.

So when you think about quitting, you think that you will lose something precious and irreplaceable rather than getting rid of an unwelcome intruder who stresses you out and makes you miserable.

> Smoking is a complete misunderstanding. All
> you are doing when you smoke it trying to get
> rid of Nitch. But by smoking you are keeping
> him alive.

quitting can be easy!

As we saw in Chapter 1, almost everyone knows the hard ways of
giving up smoking. Many people have tried them already, and most
of them have failed. The easy ways are less well known, although
hundreds of thousands of people stumble on them accidentally.

Stopping smoking is simply a matter of killing Nitch off once and
for all. By smoking, you get rid of him for a little while. By quitting
you get rid of him for ever.

But before you kill him you need to understand how he gets
your mind to play tricks on itself. You need to rid yourself of his
propaganda. If you win the propaganda war, the rest is easy. Most
quit attempts fail because the attempt is made despite continuing to
believe in his propaganda. Remember our seesaw? In white knuckle
quitting the focus is on reasons for stopping. So people write lists of
all the terrible things about smoking to increase their motivation.
But they still believe in all the benefits and pleasures of smoking. As
a result, when they quit, they believe that they are depriving
themselves of something they really want and need. Unless you see
through Nitch's propaganda, you will feel miserable, deprived and
scared. Which is exactly how Nitch wants you to feel, because he
needs you to start smoking again.

Nitch has wormed his way deep into your mind and can maintain
a running commentary whose sole purpose is to keep you smoking.

- I can't live without smoking.
- I would never be able to work properly.
- Quitting is too hard.
- I will be deprived of all the things I currently enjoy.
- A little of what you fancy does you good.
- I'll quit tomorrow.
- I could get run over by a bus tomorrow.
- It's my only pleasure.
- It takes my mind off all my problems.
- I'll never be able to relax again.
- Once a smoker always a smoker.
- It won't happen to me.
- The money isn't important.
- Who wants to be some sort of health nut anyway?
- I deserve a treat.

and so on and so on…

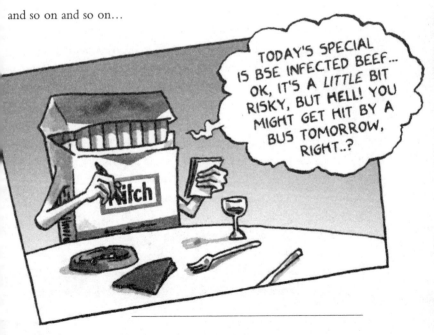

This book will help you to develop a new understanding of smoking. It will help you to explode the myths about cigarettes and expose smoking for what it really is. Cigarettes cause anxiety. They impair concentration and are a huge distraction. They destroy confidence and self-esteem. And they taste awful too!

Key Concept

Smoking gets rid of Nitch for a while.
Quitting gets rid of Nitch for ever.

chapter summary

- Being a nicotine addict can be seen as being infected with Nitch.

- Nitch has two weapons:
- The ability to make you anxious by giving you withdrawal symptoms.
- Propaganda to distort your beliefs and attitudes to smoking to make sure you keep smoking.

- Nitch gets away with this because:
- We don't recognise that he makes us anxious.
- We are looking for excuses to justify our smoking.

How Does It All Start? Addiction!

Is nicotine really addictive? And does that mean you are a drug addict? Yes and yes! Even the tobacco companies have known that nicotine is addictive since at least the 1960s, despite their continued attempts to deny this publicly. This is revealed in a series of internal documents anonymously leaked and published in 1995.[9] In an internal paper in 1963, the vice-president of Brown & Williamson Tobacco Corporation (BW), which is owned by the British American Tobacco Company (BAT), writes: 'Nicotine is addictive, we are therefore in the business of selling nicotine, an addictive drug.'[10]

BAT and BW have also known since at least the 1970s that smoking 'light' cigarettes is completely ineffective at reducing the risks of smoking because smokers will automatically take more or deeper drags in order to regulate administration of nicotine. 'Whatever the characteristics of cigarettes...the smoker adjusts his pattern to deliver his own nicotine requirements.'[11] Filtered cigarettes were also known to be ineffective for the same reason. 'The smoker of a filter cigarette was getting as much or more nicotine and tar as he would have done from a regular cigarette.'[12]

The US Surgeon General was slower to recognise this than the tobacco industry, and even today many smokers believe that switching to a 'light' or low nicotine brand is an effective way of reducing their risk – a misconception that the tobacco industry has exploited effectively through advertising. For example the advert for True Cigarettes in 1975 ran: 'All the fuss about smoking got me thinking I'd either quit, or I'd smoke True. I smoke True.'

Behaviours get the label of addictions when the costs of continuing the behaviour – for example, disease, death, financial ruin, self disgust and shame – clearly outweigh the pleasures and benefits. Some people feel uncomfortable about putting smokers in this category because smoking is so widespread and acceptable.

But history has shown that nicotine has been consumed compulsively in nearly every culture into which tobacco has been introduced. On the other hand, every nicotine-free cigarette that has ever been marketed has been a complete commercial failure.

Historical accounts also show the extreme lengths people will go to so that they can smoke. For example, during the occupation in Holland in the Second World War there was widespread starvation in many cities but nonetheless many people chose to grow tobacco instead of food, and in concentration camps cigarettes were often exchanged for food. In post-war Europe people stole and prostituted themselves in order to obtain tobacco. And in case you were in any further doubt about the power of nicotine addiction, Murad the Cruel of Turkey (1609–40) had smokers beheaded, hanged and quartered. In Romania smokers were flogged and exiled to Siberia, while in Japan in 1616 smokers were imprisoned and had their property confiscated. None of these measures stopped people smoking!

Consider the following facts:

- 92% of GPs believe that nicotine is powerfully addictive, half believing it to be more addictive than heroin or cocaine.
- 30% of smokers try to quit every year, but only 2-3% succeed.
- 60% of smokers smoke after a heart attack, 40% of them within forty-eight hours!
- 50% of smokers smoke again after surgery to remove their larynx.

- 50% of smokers smoke again after surgery to remove sections of lung.
- 80% of pregnant smokers continue to smoke throughout pregnancy.

Key Concept

Nicotine is one of the most addictive substances on Earth.

Believe it or not, cigarettes are so addictive that research has shown that over 90% of teenagers who smoke four cigarettes become regular smokers, and that the vast majority of these smokers will smoke for the rest of their lives.[13] That's all it takes. A lifetime of misery, cost and ill health for the sake of four measly cigarettes. And the worst irony of all is that those kids don't even *enjoy* those first four life-wrecking cigarettes.

It seems hard to understand, but pleasure and addiction have nothing to do with one another. Smoking is addictive. Cigarettes are addictive. That means the first cigarette you ever smoke is addictive. The confusion arises because people do not really understand how addiction works.

A defining feature of addiction is so-called compulsive use. In other words, you feel that you cannot do without whatever it is you are addicted to. So you might think that if you do not enjoy something, then you could easily do without it. If you could easily do without it, then you cannot be addicted. You are therefore safe to continue 'experimenting' or impressing your friends or whatever else it is you think you are doing. While you are not really enjoying it, it cannot be dangerous. Right?

This would seem to make sense, but unfortunately this logic is wrong. If it were true, then no one would ever get hooked. Cigarettes do not politely tap you on the shoulder and say, 'Excuse me, you have hated the taste of me so far, but the next cigarette will be like nectar from heaven and once you have tasted it you will never be able to give me up.' The first cigarette tastes bad, the fifth cigarette tastes bad and the fifty-thousandth cigarette tastes bad. Addiction has nothing to do with taste or pleasure.

so what is really going on?

When you first smoke as a youngster, you have no nicotine in your body. You therefore have no Nitch. The first cigarette puts nicotine into your body. As the nicotine leaves, you are left feeling a tiny bit stressed. Nicotine withdrawal is unpleasant from the day you start smoking, but the effects are tiny at first. Think of nicotine like paint stripper. Except instead of dissolving paint, nicotine dissolves good feelings. And as it leaves your body it takes those good feelings with it. When you smoke your second cigarette two things happen:

> 1 The toxins in the cigarette make you cough or feel sick and you experience the cigarette as horrible, just like the first one.
> 2 *At the same time*, the good feelings that the last cigarette dissolved away are restored.

Then you put out your second cigarette, and nicotine leaves your body, taking with it good feelings and leaving you feeling very slightly anxious.

What makes nicotine addiction so confusing is that nicotine withdrawal is so subtle. No two smokers describe exactly the same thing, and the symptoms that are described tend to be vague psychological-ish ones like irritability and tension. This has led some smoking cessation advisers to conclude that nicotine withdrawal is almost entirely psychological. This is wrong. Nicotine withdrawal is no less real just because it manifests itself in vague psychological or mental ways rather than with clear physiological or bodily reactions like the 'cold turkey' seen in heroin withdrawal.

Alternatively, advisers suggest that nicotine withdrawal is trivial because it is no more than mild anxiety. This is a misunderstanding. Even if anxiety is mild, people find it distressing and they are extremely motivated to reduce it. Even though anxiety is not painful or harmful, people have a strong desire to get rid of it.

As we saw in Chapter 3, anxiety is helpful. In fact it is essential for our survival, as we equate anxiety with danger. When our ancestors were out chasing woolly bears to eat, anxiety was useful. When we are walking along a steep ridge with a big drop on either side, anxiety is useful. When we are confronted by a hissing cobra, anxiety is useful. But what happens when our bodies get confused, and when anxiety symptoms are triggered in situations where they are not useful? Remember, anxiety is a biological response. Your body is not rationally weighing up the reasonableness of anxiety – it is just reacting.

With nicotine withdrawal the danger signal is chemically induced and entirely artificial. So it is not remotely useful to you. In effect your danger signal is malfunctioning and danger warnings are flashing every time you run low on nicotine. You can tell yourself logically that there is nothing to worry about – but the biological anxiety system is not logical. Your biological systems cannot tell the difference between useful anxiety that alerts us to danger, and useless anxiety that serves no purpose. It all feels the same – the drive is still to reduce it by whatever means possible.

And you have learned that smoking gets rid of it. But in fact all you have done by smoking is to reset a faulty signal, so it will go off again next time you are in the same situation.

So what can you do differently?

> • You need to unlearn that smoking is the right thing to do.
> • You need to allow the danger signal to burn itself out, and gradually fade away. If you were hungry and you ignored hunger signals you would get more and more hungry until you were starving. Eventually you would die. But if you ignore faulty anxiety signals, at first the anxiety will also get worse and worse, but gradually it will dawn on your subconscious mind that nothing bad is happening to you and anxiety will fade away and disappear.

You cannot talk yourself out of anxiety. It is not responsive to reassurance. All you can do is use logical reasoning to make sure you understand that the only way to free yourself from smoking is to override the danger signal. But you *will* feel anxious. You will have to go through a process of nicotine withdrawal to get over smoking. You need to allow yourself to go through the anxiety instead of getting rid of it, so that you can correct the faulty danger signals.

This process is *temporary*. At the end of it you will be completely free of nicotine. Any residual 'cravings' will then just be psychological – Chapter 6 addresses this.

Key Concept

Nicotine withdrawal is a short-term process. If you ignore the desire to smoke, nicotine will leave your body within a few days.

The anxiety symptoms themselves are not painful, or even particularly unpleasant. In extreme sports people use the thrill of the anxiety symptoms to have fun, to override danger signals for kicks. In bungee jumping you know perfectly well that you are securely tied to the cord and that you cannot fall, but this knowledge makes no difference to your biological anxiety response.

This is why you will still experience a compulsion to smoke, despite all logical explanations of what is happening. This is also why Nicotine Replacement Therapy (NRT), such as patches, can help, as it takes the edge off this anxiety, while you go through the task of removing the psychological dependence and the habitual aspects of smoking. (Chapter 9 provides much more information about NRT.)

Key Concept

Anxiety symptoms may be mild and vague, but we are powerfully motivated to get rid of them.

People are wrong about not getting hooked in the first place. They are also wrong time and time again about not getting re-addicted after quitting for a while. Many smokers who have experienced the misery of being hooked think, 'It won't happen again, this time I will stay in control.'

You were never in control in the first place! If you are to have any chance of lifelong quitting you need to get rid of the idea that smoking is somehow controllable and that this time you can handle it. You can't. Later chapters deal with the issue of so-called social smoking. If this is your goal, go straight to Chapter 14 and read it. If, after reading it, social smoking is still your goal then clearly you don't believe what I'm saying! If that is the case, you needn't just take my word for it. Try social smoking for yourself if you must, then when you fail and are smoking more than ever, come back and read these chapters again…

Key Concept

Nicotine withdrawal causes anxiety. To withdraw successfully from nicotine you need to override the danger signal, and ignore the powerful drive to reduce anxiety.

If you keep smoking you will reset the danger signal and anxiety will keep coming back.

taking up smoking

The most common reason for people to take up smoking is by experimenting in childhood or adolescence. Young people may be tempted to try smoking to impress their friends, out of curiosity, to rebel against parents or because they see other people smoking and believe it is enjoyable. Peer pressure is also very important. There are, however, some people who do not take up smoking until later in life.

adult experimentation

Some people start smoking at college, university, or later in life because close friends or partners smoke. This usually either stems from a desire to be sociable or happens because even non-smokers believe that smoking has benefits. If you are feeling stressed, it is natural to turn to something you think might help you. If you know anyone who is currently a non-smoker but asks you in a crisis for a cigarette, the kindest (and most honest) approach is to explain that smoking can't reduce stress in non-hooked people. And getting hooked is not going to help stress levels either.

drug use

Becoming addicted to nicotine is a physical process. So if you smoke cannabis and mix the cannabis with tobacco then you will get hooked on the nicotine in the tobacco. This happens even if you have never had any interest in smoking cigarettes, and even if you are only smoking because you like the effects of cannabis.

It may take a while to realise you are hooked, and most drug users believe that it is the cannabis they are getting hooked on, when they start craving joints. The penny usually drops when someone is running low on cannabis and starts rolling ever weaker joints, until they are actually just rolling tobacco. They then discover that the cannabis-free 'joint' does them very nicely thank-you. The message from this is that when you stop smoking, you need to stop every form of nicotine use.

the solution

You need to reset the faulty danger signal by killing Nitch. But first you need to understand his other weapon: **propaganda**, which causes psychological dependence. This is discussed in the next chapter.

chapter summary

- Nitch's first weapon is anxiety. He uses anxiety to push us around.

- The anxiety is vague but our unconscious mind sees it as a danger signal.

- We are therefore powerfully motivated to get rid of it – so we feel driven to smoke.

- Stopping smoking will allow this faulty signal to fade away.

- This should then be the end of the problem; but the misunderstanding about why we are driven to smoke gives Nitch a second weapon – propaganda.

Worksheet

ANSWER THE FOLLOWING QUESTIONS IN AS MUCH DETAIL AS POSSIBLE.

1 When did you start to smoke?

2 What were the first cigarettes like?

3 Did you believe you could get hooked?

4 If someone had asked you ten years ago if you would still be smoking today, what would you have said?

Free Yourself From Smoking

5 Have you ever tried to quit before?

6 Have you ever succeeded in quitting for longer than a few weeks?

7 If so, when you started again did you think you were 'in control' this time?

What do the answers to the above questions tell you about nicotine addiction?

The Second
Weapon: Propaganda

Nitch can physically stress you out. But he can do a lot more than that. Nitch can get into your head and tell you stuff about smoking that simply is not true. How does he get away with it?

In Chapter 3 we talked about Nitch creating anxiety whenever his nicotine levels ran a little low. This anxiety triggers a powerful drive to smoke, because the unconscious believes that the anxiety means you are in danger and directs you to reduce the anxiety (and therefore the danger) by smoking. But smokers have absolutely no idea that they are smoking in response to a biological drive. I call this the **fundamental misconception**. It has two stages:

1 Smokers notice they are relieved but do not realise that it was Nitch who was making them anxious in the first place.

2 The feeling of relief is so subtle that it does not seem important enough to explain a behaviour that is as devastating and expensive as smoking.

The apparent benefits of smoking seem so clear because anxiety levels are reduced immediately by smoking, whereas anxiety levels only increase slowly when you are not smoking. This means that a) you don't notice this pattern, and b) even if you did, it is impossible to tell that it is to do with the last cigarette you smoked. People therefore have no idea why they really smoke. But they are well aware that they do, even though they don't understand why. So they are in a state of conflict. After all, what are the experiences of a nicotine addict?

- The unpleasant taste of tobacco
- The horrid sensations of inhaling smoke
- The relief of mild anxiety (too mild to be a particularly big deal)
- The knowledge of the dangerousness of smoking
- The expense of smoking

and

- The powerful drive to smoke

Smokers therefore make sense of their powerful drive to smoke by subconsciously inventing reasons to explain the behaviour, which then develop into positive beliefs.

Key Concept

Smokers don't understand the drive to smoke, so they develop positive beliefs about smoking that provide an explanation.

Unfortunately these beliefs then make people feel deprived if they quit. To quit successfully, you need to change your internal tapes and develop a new way of thinking about cigarettes and smoking.

propaganda

When people find themselves behaving in ways they don't like, they feel extremely uncomfortable. This is known as cognitive dissonance, a state where people have conflicting thoughts about something. To reduce the discomfort, people are highly motivated to find justifications for the behaviour. They want to find excuses that make the behaviour seem okay. These excuses are not necessarily a reflection of reality. In this game, the truth doesn't matter – it's how the beliefs make you feel that count.

Key Concept

People need to be able to justify their own behaviour. If they don't know the real reasons they will invent some! This is not a conscious process.

My area of specialism within clinical psychology is Cognitive Behaviour Therapy (CBT), which has been extremely successful in highlighting and exploring the links between thoughts and feelings. People tend to think that their own thoughts are accurate reflections of the world around them. In our own minds our thoughts are intuitively and self-evidently true, whereas in fact our thinking can be highly distorted, and a million miles away from external reality.

We do not simply passively receive and process information and then make up our minds about what to think and feel. We actively construct our own worlds. For example, we see what we want and expect to see. We pay close attention to things that fit with our existing views, and tend to disregard information that contradicts those views. A good example of this is how sports fans view refereeing decisions. Decisions that go against their team are seen as outrageous and biased, while decisions that go against the opposition are seen as just and fair. (Though strangely this never happens to my team, who are always hard done by....)

Key Concept

We all actively construct our world. We quite literally see what we want and expect to see.

So what does this have to do with smoking? A simple example of how this affects smoking is to compare how afraid you are of smoking in different contexts. If you are in a pub, surrounded by other smokers, it is easy to dismiss fears of the health risks of smoking. If you are outside a hospital having a swift smoke before your appointment with a cancer doctor, fears are much harder to dismiss. The reality of the damage you are doing to yourself doesn't change. What changes is *how you feel* about that reality and even *what you believe* about that reality. Some people will readily accept that smoking is doing them serious physical harm when they are sitting in a GP's surgery being given clear information about the dangers of smoking. But later on the same day they will be throwing doubt on that information when they are with other smoking friends:

• What do doctors know? They are always getting things wrong.
• Most doctors smoke like chimneys, so who are they to tell me what to do?
• Doctors are just doom merchants, they say everything is bad for you. And they keep changing their minds anyway.

There is research evidence that clearly shows the effects of cognitive dissonance on beliefs and attitudes to smoking. For example, people who have not yet tried to quit are *more* concerned about the health consequences than people who have made a past quit attempt and failed. Why? Because people who have failed to quit experience more cognitive dissonance than people who still believe they can quit.

Smokers who have never tried to quit have the thoughts 'Smoking causes cancer' and 'I smoke'. This creates dissonance. How can this dissonance be reduced? Well, one way is to develop a third thought, which is 'I'll quit some time'.

But people who have tried to quit don't have the luxury of this third thought. Instead they have the thoughts 'Smoking causes cancer', 'I smoke' and 'I can't stop smoking'. This creates greater dissonance, which must be reduced, and the only way is to change their attitudes about the first thought – the health costs. If you have greater amounts of cognitive dissonance you have to go to greater lengths to reduce it by denying that the costs of smoking are real or relevant. This is not rational. But it is what most smokers do. This process is not conscious. It happens totally automatically and you probably do it too!

thinking errors

What I call thinking errors refers to thoughts that are in some way inaccurate, distorted or biased, and are how we solve our problems of cognitive dissonance. Having different thoughts about how dangerous smoking is in different situations is one example of distorting or denying reality. There are many types of thinking error.

minimisation

This is typified by the 'Don't worry, be happy' frame of mind. Minimising means playing down the consequences of smoking, for example telling yourself that you've got to die some time, or that serious illnesses don't worry you, or that money is irrelevant, or that you wouldn't want to live for ever anyway.

It is important to remember that the distorted thoughts you have about smoking won't seem distorted to you – they will seem entirely plausible and self-evidently true! So you must be ruthlessly honest with yourself. Don't accept your own thinking and rationalising at face value.

Smokers die an average of sixteen years early. *Sixteen years!* Think of someone you know who has died of a smoking-related disease. What would sixteen extra years have meant to them, to you, to their families? Think of an elderly non-smoker who died. Imagine losing the last sixteen years with them. How much precious life would they have missed?

Many people minimise smoking. This is not because smokers are happy-go-lucky, laid-back people. Even smokers who think they are realistic about the dangers are more than likely kidding themselves. They might believe it intellectually, but this knowledge has little emotional impact. When I smoked I believed virtually everyone who smoked died of it in the end. Then I read that in fact one in four smokers died from smoking (as was thought at that time). I was genuinely happy about this! I thought that those odds were pretty good so I could stop worrying about it.

If you are thinking, 'Well, those *are* good odds,' contrast that with concern about AIDS or BSE. People become terribly worried about contracting these awful diseases, but the odds against dying of them are many thousands to one. With smoking the odds are 50:50! Smokers have to insulate themselves from the dangers of smoking, because otherwise the cognitive dissonance would be too high to bear.

Minimising the financial costs is also very common. But this does not mean smokers are more generous than average and are happy to throw their money around. When smokers say money isn't important they are usually referring exclusively to money for cigarettes. They are not saying they would be happy to pay over the odds for their shopping, or for petrol, or for insurance, or for holidays abroad, or indeed for anything at all except smoking. So money is important in every other area of life. It is not them who don't mind the money – it's Nitch who doesn't think the money is important. But then he's not the one spending it!

denial

Denial, or the 'ostrich syndrome', is similar to minimisation, but takes it a step further. Rather than thinking, 'Well it might happen, but so what?', people in denial simply assume that it will not happen to them. Smokers receive large amounts of smoking-related information from a variety of sources. These include doctors, magazines, newspapers, advertisements, personal experience, conversations with other people, television images, books and so on. If we were entirely rational beings we would treat all incoming material equally. We would register the information, assess the reliability of the source and make a balanced judgement about how credible or true this information is. Of course we do no such thing.

In the first place we usually notice or seek out information that fits with what we already believe. If we are given information that we don't like, we just ignore it. Thoughts include:

- They say everything gives you cancer these days.
- If I didn't smoke I'd be more stressed so my health would suffer.
- My uncle lived to eighty and he smoked two packs a day.
- Statistics don't mean anything.
- I eat well and exercise so I'm pretty healthy really.
- I don't inhale.
- I only smoke menthols.
- Loads of people smoke so it can't be that bad.
- My aunt gave up smoking and developed pneumonia.

In 1964 when the US Surgeon General first published links between smoking and cancer, some research was done on how this information was viewed by the public. Only 10% of non-smokers thought the evidence for links between smoking and cancer was flawed, compared with 40% of smokers. In other words we often believe what we want to believe rather than making a rational judgement on the basis of the evidence. Cognitive dissonance turns us from rational beings into rationalising beings.

Key Concept

Cognitive dissonance turns us from rational beings into rationalising beings.

You may have seen a programme on television about an expensive health farm. Part of the weekly programme involved a quitting smoking package. A quitter in his thirties was having a medical examination. This involved blowing into a tube to test his lung function. The other smokers were standing around waiting for their turn and the atmosphere was relaxed.

'Well, Mr Smith, let's see how your bellows are doing,' says the physiologist cheerfully. After the test he tut-tuts and says, 'Oh dear...' in mock disapproval. Giggles all round. 'Mr Smith, your lungs are about twenty years older than the rest of you!' Mr Smith pulls an 'Oops, silly me' kind of a face and grins ruefully. The rest of the group giggles.

This was not fiction but real people on a real course. The amazing thing about this scene is how totally inappropriate everybody's emotional responses are. Imagine anyone being given similarly devastating medical information in any other context: a diabetic being told his kidneys were packing up or a miner that he had lung damage.

Any time people are exposed to dangerous substances such as asbestos or silicon they become (quite reasonably) extremely anxious. If subsequent tests show damage the response is fear, anger and disbelief.

But when it comes to damage due to smoking, people treat it like some big joke. This is a classic example of the ostrich syndrome. Smokers ignore and dismiss any scary information, either refusing to believe the dangers, or refusing to think realistically about their implications. This is one reason why shock tactics rarely work.

rose-tinted glasses

Just as we downplay the costs and risks of smoking, so we exaggerate the benefits and put cigarettes on a pedestal. Even cigarettes that are actually a downright pain in the neck to smoke – because of the circumstances in which we smoke them – tend to be viewed positively.

arbitrary inference

Arbitrary inference refers to the fact that we are not very good scientists. A scientist makes careful, unbiased observations and then draws conclusions from them. Most people, however, jump to conclusions on far more flimsy evidence. If we see a smoker who looks fit and healthy we tend to think, 'Well, he seems fine, so smoking can't be that bad.' Or happy, smiley smokers make us think that smoking is relaxing, pleasant and fun. Yet when we see miserable-looking people smoking we tend to blame their misery on the fact that they are probably homeless, or that it's raining, or that it is Monday morning and they are on their way to work – it never crosses our mind that they might be miserable because they smoke.

Free Yourself From Smoking

selective attention

This refers to the fact that we do not observe the world in a consistent way. We notice some things far more than others, even if both are equally visible. In other words, our perception is influenced by our current concerns. An example of this is the way that when women become pregnant the world suddenly seems full of other pregnant women. Or that when you learn a new word you start seeing it everywhere. Selective attention also affects smokers. When you are struggling to cope without cigarettes the world suddenly seems full of relaxed and happy smokers! In truth, smokers are more miserable, stressed and tense than non-smokers. If your observations tell you different, that's just because you are observing the things you expect to see and failing to notice other evidence.

Try to reverse this tendency. Next time you are out, carefully watch all smokers. Not just the handsome, fit, healthy, happy-looking ones, but the coughing, grumpy, wrinkled miserable ones too.

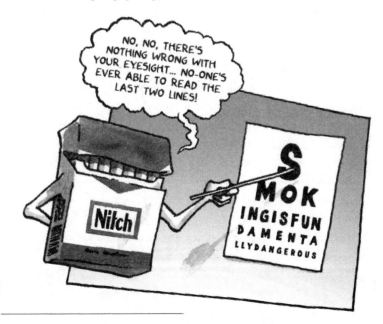

inevitability

Some people think that they have no option but to smoke. So they might as well make the best of it. 'I'm an addict,' they say. But this does not condemn them to a lifetime of smoking. Everyone who has ever smoked in the past was an addict for as long as they continued to smoke. And millions have successfully quit. Telling yourself that you have no choice is a cop out. Don't let yourself off the hook like that. Yes, you are an addict. But you can stop smoking anyhow.

deal-making/bargaining

When people want something they don't think they should have, they sometimes try to bargain with themselves. In fact some people use bargaining or deal-making to persuade themselves to stop smoking in the first place. Once, when I was still a smoker, I realised that I was sick of feeling tired and unhealthy, so I decided to quit smoking and get fit. I started jogging and quickly noticed that I could go a little further every day. This evidence of success was powerfully motivating and for a while my quit attempt went really well.

Unfortunately I hadn't got rid of any of the positive beliefs about smoking. I thought that I was making a big sacrifice for the sake of my health and, though I was pleased with my progress, I still missed cigarettes. After a while, the nicotine withdrawal was over, and so I should have been free. But I wasn't, because I still thought of cigarettes in a positive way. Gradually I got used to the fact that I could run, and it stopped being such a good motivator. I was glad to be fitter but it wasn't such a big deal any more. The desire for a cigarette began to outweigh the desire to stay stopped. I started thinking, 'Well, I can run four miles now, that'll do. I mean, how fit do I want to be?'

Eventually I made a deal with myself. I was allowed to smoke again, but only after I had exercised that day. In that way I was going to keep fit but still be allowed to smoke. Excellent plan! I even told myself that

I would be healthier that way, because any damage done by smoking would be cancelled out by running. I was a medical student at the time and knew that this was utter rubbish. However healthy taking exercise may be, it does not cancel out the effects of smoking. But smokers do not let inconvenient things like reality get in the way of smoking, so I spent the next week or so only smoking after I had been running.

Soon enough the day came when it was raining and I couldn't be bothered to run. But I wanted to smoke. I was totally back into smoking and couldn't imagine not having a cigarette. So I leapt to my feet, did ten star jumps and then lit up, thinking, 'Well, I've done my exercise so that's okay.'

This episode shows the problem with bargaining. If you have done quite well in stopping smoking, just having the odd one seems possible, and any deal that lets you smoke occasionally seems quite good. But as soon as you are smoking regularly, Nitch has got his claws well and truly into you again, and whatever bargain you originally made won't ever seem enough. Nitch cannot be bargained with. He'll say absolutely anything to get that first post-quitting fag lit, then go back on the deal. As soon as he gets his foot in the door he will be prising it wide open. So do not kid yourself with the false promise of deals and bargains.

catastrophisation

This thinking error involves believing the worst about a situation. For a smoker, this might be thoughts like 'If I quit I will never be happy again' or 'Smoking is my best friend, it's all I've got left'.

This sort of statement can feel very powerful, but is usually grossly exaggerated. No one is 'never happy again', despite dreadful hardships. Just take a look around the world and don't exaggerate your difficulties. Quitting is a period of adjustment, following which you will still be you, enjoying the things you enjoy, seeing the people you like to see, doing the things you like to do.

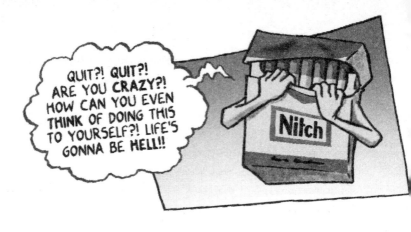

One of the key features of thinking errors is that thoughts feel true to the person having them, no matter how far-fetched. If we say to ourselves, 'I'll never be happy again' or 'Everyone hates me' or 'If I fail to get this job I'm a worthless person and I'll never succeed in life', these thoughts are exaggerated. But we respond emotionally to them as if they were true. We don't have 'exaggeration filters' between our thoughts and our feelings. If we think it we feel it. So make sure you don't allow your thoughts to be extreme, exaggerated or catastrophic. Take a bit of a reality check every so often.

As for 'Smoking is all I have' – well, if this is true then you seriously need to quit! Most smokers who describe their smoking as their 'best friend' or 'only pleasure' have many friends and family (who may be somewhat offended to think that you consider them irrelevant!). Be honest about the things of value in your life. Who do you care about, who cares about you, what do you like doing? Do not give cigarettes status that they do not deserve.

If you really feel very lonely and you do not have any activities that you enjoy, then this is a problem in its own right. You need to try to deal with that problem at the same time as quitting. Smoking is not helping you to make friends and develop social activities. All it is doing is costing you money that you could use far more effectively by joining a club or group or activity, and costing you health, which will make it even harder to get out and about.

Another example of catastrophic thinking is that stopping smoking will prevent you from working. Many people use this as an excuse to continue smoking, believing that if they quit they will be unable to function. This is also inaccurate. It may be true that when King George V was operated on, his surgeon puffed over the anaesthetised body, but surgeons nowadays are not allowed to smoke in operating theatres. And yet they can carry out many hours of intensely concentrated work, without smoking – even the ones who are heavy smokers. Surgeons who smoke will come out of theatre after a four-hour operation and immediately light up. They may at that point believe that they need that cigarette. But if the operation took five, six or seven hours they would have had no problem staying focused. You do not need cigarettes to do your job.

selective memory

This refers to the human tendency to remember things in a biased way. Research has shown that what we can remember depends on factors such as mood, situation and beliefs. If we are happy, we tend to remember other times when we were happy. If we are sad, we remember sad times. When people quit smoking, they remember cigarettes in a biased way. Most cigarettes are smoked automatically and are not pleasurable. Some cigarettes are actively horrible. But when we quit we forget all about those ones. Instead we remember the 'good' cigarettes, such as smokes we had after a long period of not smoking.

In a similar way, when we have relapsed after a period of quitting, we forget that quitting wasn't that bad. This is a strange mental trick that you are more likely to notice in other people than in yourself – because you won't remember it for yourself. But, believe me, you probably do it.

A friend of mine recently quit smoking. For the first three weeks he was fine. He was positive, determined and motivated. For the next four months he continued not to smoke and carried on feeling fine about it. He told me he was really pleased he had stopped and would never go back to smoking again. A week later I saw him lighting up in the pub. He told me he was 'just having the odd one', because he had overcome the addiction and would never go back to regular smoking. I knew he was sunk at that point, but I rarely talk to people about smoking unless they ask for my advice, so I just sadly watched as his 'occasional cigarettes' became more and more frequent. Finally a few weeks later he bought a packet from the pub machine. He lit up with a sigh of pure rapture, looked lovingly at the glowing end of his fag and said, 'Thank goodness I'm smoking again after four months of torture.'

It is important to recognise that he was not deliberately lying. He truly believed his four months' abstinence had been terrible, because as a (re)addicted smoker he could not imagine life without smoking. But in reality he had been absolutely fine.

co-collusion

This refers to the way smokers talk about smoking to each other. Nitch's propaganda is triply powerful because there are millions of smokers all with their own little parasitic Nitches, all being fed propaganda and all believing it. So your own beliefs are echoed again and again by other people. In addition smokers will try to support the inaccurate beliefs of other smokers, in the hope that the other smoker will do the same for them. Smokers need to feel better about their smoking. So if Smoker A makes Smoker B feel better, then Smoker B will make Smoker A feel better in return.

This is illustrated in the following conversation:

'I saw my doctor today. He told me to quit smoking.'
'Don't they always?'
'My chest feels a bit rubbish. But it's only a cold.'
'Doctors drive me mad. They never let smokers get colds or coughs – it is always blamed on smoking.'
'I reckon I get fewer colds than non-smokers I know.'
'Me too. I've always thought germs couldn't survive in my lungs. I smoke 'em out.' (Laughs.)
'Double vodkas do the same thing for my stomach! Drink?'
'Double vodka sounds good. Fag?'
'Cheers, mate.'

Key Concept

> Smokers make many thinking errors' about their smoking. These errors make them less likely to quit and more likely to be miserable if they do quit.

why do people make thinking errors?

Thinking errors have different functions. Selective memory and denial serve the function of protecting you, the smoker, from the dreadful realities of smoking. Or, rather, they protect you from thinking about them – you are still (unfortunately) living the terrible realities.

No one intends or wants to keep smoking for life. They always believe quitting will be in the fairly near (but not too near) future. People often despair when the realisation dawns that they are actually hooked on these horrible things. The 'head in the sand' attitude can make a rapid reappearance under these circumstances.

I had a friend at university who smoked. She always said she felt fine about her smoking because she enjoyed it and because it helped her cope with the stresses of her course. However, she did not see herself as a smoking forty-year-old. Smoking was fine, for now, but would not be a habit she continued for much longer. She consistently said that she would stop after her final-year exams. This reassuring belief meant that she could smoke without worrying too much about it, safe in the knowledge that she was going to quit quite soon.

Several months after the exams I met her at a party. Surprise, surprise, she was smoking.

'What happened to quitting?' I asked.

'Oh, I never intended to quit, I like smoking,' she replied.

Now she wasn't lying. She honestly believed that she never intended to quit. Because if she wanted to quit but couldn't, what would that mean? If she couldn't quit, now, today, why would she be able to quit tomorrow or the next day or the day after that?

This reality was so uncomfortable that my friend genuinely erased her plans to quit from memory. When it came to it she felt she could not quit. She did not want to admit that she was hopelessly hooked and so clung to a belief that smoking was a choice: she was smoking because she enjoyed it. Her memory then edited out evidence that smoking was not a choice.

Some thinking errors make you believe you need cigarettes, for example, catastrophisation and putting cigarettes on a pedestal. All the errors can be viewed as 'propaganda' peddled by Nitch to make you carry on smoking.

propaganda and quitting

Let's look at the process of quitting again. People tend to focus on their feelings and assume that their thoughts stem from their feelings. For example:

FEELINGS: misery when I try to stop smoking, results in
THOUGHTS: I need to smoke or I will be miserable.

In reality the process works the other way around. Thoughts drive feelings, not vice versa. In other words:

THOUGHTS: I need cigarettes or I will be miserable, leads to
FEELINGS: misery when I don't smoke.

If you change the message in your head the feelings change too. This is why the same smoker can have different quit experiences if the thoughts are different each time.

Key Concept

Thoughts often drive feelings, not the other way around.

The misery of quitting is not caused by withdrawal symptoms but by the exhausting running commentary in your head: 'Go on, have one, just one won't hurt, you deserve a treat.' So how can you change the internal tape? Well, you need to understand how Nitch operates. If you understand the process you can disarm it. Nitch peddles this nonsense about smoking because his entire existence depends on you lighting up the next cigarette. Imagine an alcoholic who thinks, 'Drink gives me courage and confidence.' It is obvious to everyone that drink is sapping his courage and confidence, but the alcoholic clings to a belief that is clearly untrue, to justify carrying on drinking. Addicted thinking is faulty thinking and smokers are just as deluded as any other addicts.

Key Concept

Addicted thinking is faulty thinking.

So how can Nitch make us believe all this rubbish if it isn't true? Why is it so easy for him to fool us for so long?

I don't like feeling stupid!

As we have seen, cognitive dissonance is very uncomfortable and the more smoking affects us, the more we need to find reasons to explain why we smoke, and to justify it to ourselves. If you are smoking now, the odds are against you ever stopping no matter what the cost. The vast majority of smokers smoke for life.

Almost everyone hopes and believes that they will stop one day – just never today! But the cunning nature of Nitch's trap means that as costs rise, the more you believe you need cigarettes.

Imagine the following situations:

• You are in a pub surrounded by relaxed, happy smokers. You light up. Your justification? 'It's sociable and enjoyable.' Sociability or enjoyment is enough of a reason, because the costs of smoking are not immediately obvious in that situation, so you will not be particularly worried about smoking.

- You are at a party and no one else is smoking. You go outside to light up, feeling a bit embarrassed. Your justification? 'I want to relax and smoking helps me. I won't enjoy it so much otherwise.' You need a different reason from 'enjoyment' or 'sociability' because you are not enjoying the cigarette much, and you are not being sociable.
- You are at home by yourself and you have a bad cough. You light up. Your justification? 'I'm too stressed without it.'
- You are in hospital and you crawl from your bed dragging your dripstand down the corridor to stand in the chilly doorway in your night-clothes. You light up. Your justification? 'I can't live without it.'

Your reason goes from pleasure (enjoyment) to benefit (relaxation, concentration) to need (can't live/cope without it). No matter what the situation, you feel you want or need *this* cigarette in *this* situation. So you will never give up, because no matter how bad things get for you, Nitch keeps one step ahead, making you believe you can't live without it. The problem is not the cigarette, it is the power that *you* give the cigarette. Disarm it now. Change your thinking and the cigarettes will lose their power.

Key Concept

The more you want to stop smoking, the more cognitive dissonance you have, so the more positively you view cigarettes. The desire to smoke keeps up with the desperation to quit.

chapter summary

• Nitch's second weapon is propaganda.

• Smokers do not understand the drive to smoke.

• Smokers do not really enjoy smoking.

• But smokers know smoking is deadly.

• This causes cognitive dissonance which makes smokers feel stupid and uncomfortable.

• Smokers reduce dissonance by downplaying the risks and elevating the benefits.

• The difficulties of quitting lie in the power you give the cigarette, not in qualities of the cigarettes themselves.

• A secret of successful quitting is to stop giving cigarettes so much power. The next chapter will show you how....

Free Yourself From Smoking

Worksheet

Have a look at the following common thoughts smokers have. Next to each statement, write down a counter-statement. The first one has been done for you as an example.

Statement	Counter-statement
I could get run over by a bus tomorrow.	Yes, but I probably won't, so it would make more sense to live my life and base my decisions on the assumption that this won't happen.
You can prove anything with statistics.	
I'm young. I don't care about what happens when I am older.	
My nan smoked till she was eighty-five.	

Statement	Counter-statement
I'll quit before I get ill.	
Life is too short to spend it worrying.	
It will never happen to me.	
Lots of people smoke. They aren't worried so why should I be?	
I'm not hooked. I just enjoy it. I can quit any time.	
I don't have to smoke, I choose to smoke.	

Exploding the Myths

We have learned that Nitch has two weapons: stress and propaganda. A basic message of this book is that the pleasures and benefits of smoking are actually costs in disguise. When I was a smoker, if someone had told me I didn't really enjoy smoking I imagine my reaction would have been along the lines of 'And how on earth can you claim to know how someone else experiences smoking? If I say I enjoy cigarettes and find them relaxing, then smoking is enjoyable and relaxing and who are you to tell me otherwise?'

This is a perfectly reasonable question, so I'll try to answer it by exploring the supposed pleasures and benefits in detail.

stress and relaxation

Smoking helps people relax. This 'fact' is almost universally accepted. Even non-smokers who are stressed sometimes say they wished they smoked so that they could have something to help them cope. Advice about quitting often suggests that people learn relaxation techniques so that they can get the benefit of relaxation without needing to smoke While it is helpful to learn to relax (see chapter 10), this does not mean that smoking is relaxing and therefore needs replacing. People are advised to quit during holidays or times when they are less stressed.

The 'fact' that cigarettes are relaxing is ingrained so deeply in our culture and psyche that at first it seems absurd to dispute this. 'Everyone knows' smoking calms people down. Some doctors actually recommend that people continue to smoke if they are undergoing severe stresses.

But there is not one shred of factual evidence that supports this belief.

On the contrary, there is an ever-increasing body of evidence that shows that smoking is stressful. And that does not just mean that the hardships you have to deal with if you are a smoker, such as the expense and the damage to health, are stressful. It means that smoking itself is stressful.

Key Concept

Smoking is stressful, *not* relaxing.

However, I am not suggesting for one moment that people don't feel more relaxed after a cigarette than before it. What I am saying is that people experience cigarettes as relaxing when in fact they are stressful.

Some of you may think I have lost the plot a bit here, but grasping what I have just said is absolutely crucial in understanding (and thereby freeing yourself from) smoking.

- You experience smoking as relaxing.
- You feel more relaxed after a cigarette.
- But cigarettes are stressful.

How can all these statements be true?

Consider what happens when you put out a cigarette. As we have already seen, nicotine rapidly leaves your body, and you begin to experience the effects of nicotine withdrawal. The effects vary from person to person, but most people feel stressed, tense or restless. These feelings build up very gradually over time. At first the feelings are so subtle that you barely notice them but after a while you begin to think about cigarettes again. Your body has prompted your brain to think about smoking because the tension has reached a level where it is noticed. These feelings can be summarised by the word anxiety. Anxiety triggers the thought, 'I want a cigarette.' So you have one and instantly feel relieved.

Key Concept

Cigarettes appear to be relaxing as they remove the stress that they created.

This happens again and again and again in an unbreaking chain. A cigarette causes anxiety which is relieved by a cigarette which causes anxiety which is relieved by a cigarette which causes anxiety which...on and on and on. This miserable and stressful chain can (and usually does) last a lifetime.

Unless you break it!

The real tragedy about being trapped in the smoking chain is that people forget what being relaxed actually feels like. People are so used to the ever-present stresses and aggravations of life as a smoker that they think they feel normal.

This is shown in the following diagram:

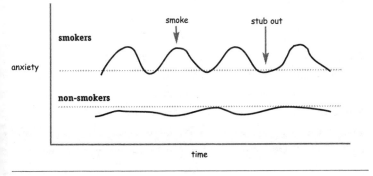

Smokers are withdrawing from nicotine *almost all the time*. Which means that they are enduring the hassle of Nitch's whingeing almost all the time. On the graph notice how the anxiety levels of the smoker rise, then drop sharply when the person smokes. This makes smoking feel satisfying. But notice that the anxiety levels for the smokers are higher all the time than those for non-smokers.

The feelings of nicotine withdrawal are so much part of smokers' lives that they become the norm. Unless smokers are actually deprived of cigarettes (when the common or garden Nitch whingeing turns into a full-blown Nitch tantrum) they go through the day feeling stressed and getting rid of the feeling without ever really being aware of how much tension cigarettes cause. They just think, 'I want a cigarette,' then they have one and think, 'That's better.'

Better than what?

Better than not having one.

And why is that?

Because not having one is a source of tension.

Imagine that you want a cigarette but are not able to have one. I'm sure that is a familiar feeling! You feel restless and unsettled and you cannot concentrate on anything. You have a persistent little voice in your head saying, 'I want to smoke,' 'I want a cigarette,' 'Where can I get some cigarettes?' That uncomfortable restless feeling is Nitch. You never had that feeling until you started to smoke. Non-smokers never have that feeling. The feeling was created when you started to smoke and is being maintained because you continue to smoke. It is an entirely artificial feeling caused by nicotine addiction. That feeling is the feeling of being a smoker. And it is horrible!

I once quit smoking using the willpower method and sweated it out for about ten weeks. It was miserable at first but over the last two to three weeks I wasn't really thinking about smoking any more and I felt confident that I had cracked it. So confident that I felt 'safe enough' to smoke a couple when I went out one night. A few days later I smoked a couple more, then more than a couple more! Finally, one Friday when we were having a quick drink after work, my friends insisted I buy my own so I bought a packet, gave a few away and then went home. I was living alone at the time. Now despite the fact that I had been smoking all week, I was still labouring under the delusion that I wasn't a smoker again. I was telling myself that I hadn't really started smoking again, I was just 'being sociable'. But now I was at home on my own with this packet of cigarettes burning a hole in my pocket. If I smoked them, I would be admitting that I was a smoker – not even I could pretend that smoking my own cigarettes, by myself in my flat, was a sociable thing to do. So I was trying to resist. Trying desperately to resist. But I really *really* wanted to smoke.

This voice in my head (aka Nitch) just would not shut up:

'Have a fag, it's a Friday night, I've had a hard week,
I deserve a treat.'
'Have a fag, I don't have much money for heaven's sake,
I can't waste them.'
'Just finish the packet and then quit again.'
'A cigarette would be lovely now, go on, I really want to.'
'Just one won't hurt. I deserve a treat. It's the evening. Why
shouldn't I just chill out and relax with a nice cigarette?'
'Plenty of people smoke, why am I making such a big deal
about it? I'll just smoke occasionally – I've already proved I
don't need to smoke all the time.'
'It's Friday night, I deserve a treat after a hard week'.

I tried to watch television but couldn't settle. I tried to read a book, but couldn't concentrate. I tried to cook a meal. But I didn't want a meal – I wanted a fag! I started pacing the living room and all the while the voice in my head continued:

> 'Have a fag, things are hard for me at the moment, I need
> something to help me.'
> 'Have a fag, why should I make myself miserable?'
> 'Have a fag, it's only a fag for goodness sake, why am I
> making such a big deal out of it?'
> 'Have a fag, have a fag, have a fag....'

In the end I suddenly thought, 'This is ridiculous. If I want it that much, then I'm just going to have it. It's only a cigarette. It's not crack cocaine. Just have the damn thing.' So I took a cigarette out of the packet and was about to light up when it suddenly struck me, in a moment of total clarity that *the only reason I wanted this cigarette was to stop myself wanting it. The only reason I wanted this cigarette was that thoughts of it had consumed me for hours and I was sick of thinking about it. The only reason I wanted to smoke was to stop myself wanting to smoke so I could actually think about or do something else that evening. But the only reason I wanted to smoke was because I had smoked the last one. And smoking this one would guarantee the need to smoke the next one, and the one after that, and the one after that.*

I realised that really wanting cigarettes was a horrible state to be in. Usually when I really want something it's because that thing is of genuine worth and value. But the desire to smoke is different. It is not a desire to do something worthwhile, or fun, or exciting, or pleasurable. It is just a desire to get rid of the desire! And it is a horrid feeling. The desire to go skiing is an exciting feeling. The desire to smoke is utterly negative.

All a cigarette does is get rid of the desire for a cigarette. But the only reason you have the desire is because of the last cigarette you smoked. Wanting to smoke feels horrible. Smoking stops you wanting to smoke for a little while. *And that is all it does.*

I sat there looking at the cigarette I was just about to light. I thought about how my evening had been dominated by thinking about smoking and I remembered how as a smoker my whole life had been dominated by the need and desire to smoke. Just a short week ago that desire was not there. And cigarettes were meaningless in my life. I realised I had a choice. Light the fag and keep the horrid feelings of needing and craving cigarettes alive, or ride out the feeling and get rid of it for good. I didn't light up.

Key Concept

All smoking does is stop you wanting to smoke – for a while.

The belief that smoking is relaxing is a **fundamental misconception** which keeps people stuck in the Smoking Triangle for smoke after smoke after smoke. The key to successful quitting is to see through it.

Imagine the scene: you have had a terrible day at work. Your boss has yelled at you. You have a thumping headache. It's pouring with rain and you don't have an umbrella. Your car is in the garage so you have to get a bus home. You sit on the bus soaking wet and cold. It lurches forward in fits and starts caught in a dreadful traffic jam. When you get home you find you have lost your keys.

You sit on the doorstep in a terrible mood and light a cigarette. Immediately you feel better. Your situation has not improved but at least you can have a fag and this helps. Someone else in an identical situation would not have the benefit of that cigarette. So you are better off – right? Wrong!

Not only did you have to contend with the bad day at work, the hassle with the boss, the headache, the rain, traffic and lost keys. On top of all this misery Nitch made an appearance too. Whining at you, demanding attention, insisting on being fed *now*! As if you didn't have enough to worry about. Think of Nitch as an annoying, persistent, ever-present little creature who won't take no for an answer. He hassles you and bugs you and irritates you until you give in and feed him – i.e. smoke. As soon as you feed him he shuts up and gives you some peace. So you experience relief – for a little while. But you are only relieving the stress that Nitch caused. Non-smokers in exactly the same position simply wouldn't have the extra hassle of having Nitch to deal with on top of all their other worries.

Key Concept

Smokers have all the real-life problems non-smokers have. On top of these they have Nitch.

I repeat: smoking is *not* relaxing; it is incredibly stressful. Even if cigarettes were harmless, just being a slave to Nitch is enormously stressful. Smokers have to accept that their addiction means that they always have to think about cigarettes. Wherever they go they need to make sure their supply doesn't run out. If they are short of money they need to make other sacrifices.

In my smoking groups a number of smokers laugh at the ridiculous idea that they would ever find themselves running short of cigarettes. Some people go pale at the thought. This neatly illustrates how conscious and aware smokers are of the need to keep themselves permanently supplied with cigarettes. But I was the type of disorganised smoker who kept running out. And what a nightmare that was! Imagine you are in a pub and suddenly discover you have only two cigarettes left. And you don't have much money. What are your options? Buy another drink, or buy some more fags?

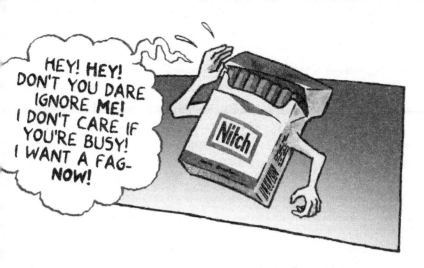

No contest! Unless you are confident of your scrounging abilities (or you are an alcoholic too) cigarettes win hands down. I once spent two hours standing on my own outside a cinema waiting for my friends. I had realised after meeting up with them that I couldn't afford both a packet of cigarettes and a cinema ticket and naturally the cigarettes won. I was only fifteen! I would never have dreamt that I could be hooked at that age. Cigarettes hook you fast.

Imagine you are on a camping trip and you get to your tent in the pouring rain to discover your cigarettes are drenched and have disintegrated. A weekend of not smoking stretches before you. How far would you be prepared to walk (in the rain) to buy some more? How many total strangers would you be prepared to ask for fags? Now imagine how you would feel asking the same strangers for food or water! When it comes to satisfying Nitch, smokers are tireless and shameless. And this endless pandering to Nitch's desires is unbelievably stressful. The best thing about quitting for me wasn't the health gains, or the extra money. It was the sheer blissful relief of never having to think about Nitch again. It was an unbelievably precious sense of freedom. Once Nitch is dead, you can be completely free of him – providing, of course, that you no longer believe his propaganda.

'But I enjoy smoking!' I hear you cry impatiently. Okay, let's look at enjoyment.

enjoyment

What do you enjoy about a cigarette? The taste? The sensation of the smoke hitting the back of your throat? The deep breath in and the steady stream of smoke you blow out? Beautifully crafted smoke rings? The feel of it in your hand – feeling so *right* there? The shiny packets lined up enticingly on the newsagent's shelves? I can still remember the tingle of anticipation I felt just seeing a shiny new packet, full of promises of comfort and luxury and indulgence.

Let's start with taste. Can you remember your first cigarette? Unless you started later in life when you had already been victim to passive smoking for a while, or unless you had used tobacco in other forms before starting to smoke cigarettes, the first cigarette would not have relieved you of any tension. If you had never had any nicotine before, you would not yet have had the misfortune of meeting Nitch.

That first experience of smoking is what a cigarette is really like. Until Nitch sets up camp in your body, all cigarettes taste terrible.

At this early stage, smoking is largely image and nothing else. So kids will claim to enjoy their first few cigarettes. This is never true. Cigarettes are horrible when you are not addicted to nicotine. Even kids seem to know this and are on the lookout for anyone who is just pretending to inhale.

When I started smoking, the girls in my class who smoked met in McDonalds every Saturday. We would immediately light up. Anyone watching would have been able to witness the ludicrous spectacle of half a dozen fourteen-year-old girls taking pathetic little drags, saying things like, 'God I need this' and trying desperately to leave the stub burning between drags so that they didn't have to smoke so much without anyone noticing.

We girls were deeply suspicious of anyone who might not really be inhaling. We would watch newcomers to the group like hawks, ready to pounce on them.

'You didn't inhale,' we would shout accusingly.

'I did, I did,' would come the plaintive cry.

'Prove it!' we would demand and the poor smoker would have to inhale, say a few words, then exhale. Only then would they have passed our stupid little test.

So what was going on there? Here was a group of teenagers all doing something they secretly knew they hated, all deeply suspicious that other people might hate it too, and all utterly contemptuous of anyone if they showed evidence that they did hate it.

Once at the weekly McDonalds trip a new girl joined us. After we had smoked the obligatory B&H we stubbed them out with relief. To our horror the new girl took another fag out of the packet, then offered the pack around. Another one – no way! But image was all-important so we all dutifully lit up again (with exclamations of gratitude). Afterwards I was sick.

Those early cigarettes represent what cigarettes truly taste like, if you don't have nicotine addiction as a complicating factor. They taste disgusting. And cigarettes don't change!

Key Concept

Cigarettes taste disgusting – you just get used to it.

Addicted smokers 'develop a taste' for cigarettes because over time they come to associate smoking with relief. The only 'good' bit about smoking is relief from nicotine withdrawal. In fact, that is the only thing that matters at all. If someone gave you a cigarette that was identical in taste and smell to your normal cigarettes, but had no nicotine in it, it would give you no satisfaction. But the fact that your cigarettes do contain nicotine means that they do satisfy.

It is therefore crucial to successful quitting to recognise that the feelings of satisfaction arise from a misconception: this happens because people confuse relief with pleasure. Relief is the removal of something unpleasant (which makes you feel better afterwards). True pleasures add something to your life. And when you also consider that the unpleasantness that is *removed* by smoking is actually *caused* by smoking, it becomes clear that there is no good reason to continue at all. Cigarettes are not enjoyable to smoke. All aspects of smoking are in themselves unpleasant. The taste and smell are unpleasant. The sensation of smoke entering your lungs is horrid. And the handling aspects are irrelevant. They only seem pleasant or important because you have become conditioned to associate these actions with relief.

But even the genuine relief is no reason to smoke, because smoking only relieves the misery it causes.

The pleasure of smoking is simply the relief of Nitch-whingeing

Which cigarettes do you 'enjoy' most? Most people find the cigarettes they smoke after a longish gap to be most satisfying. For example, the smoke after a meal, or the first one after you have been out shopping.

But all cigarettes are the same! This is so blindingly obvious but is rarely considered by smokers. All cigarettes (at least those from the same packet) are the same! The cigarette doesn't change just because it's after a meal. The difference is simply how much you need the nicotine.

The difference between pleasure and relief is shown in the following story. Years ago when I still smoked I had the incredible opportunity to go to Spitsbergen in the High Arctic for nine weeks on a mountaineering trip. I knew I couldn't smoke when I was there, because we would be completely cut off from civilisation. I was very worried about how bad the first few days/weeks would be because I had experienced terrible withdrawal cravings in my many previous failed attempts at quitting. I never intended to quit completely at that time because I believed that the only way of coping on the utterly smokeless Arctic ice cap was to think about the glorious promise of the cigarettes to come when we got back to civilisation. So just as we all coped with bland, monotonous rehydrated food by dreaming endlessly about the gorgeous feast we would have in a few weeks' time, I did exactly the same thing with cigarettes – picturing myself outside the tent, in a bar, on a mountain, dragging deeply and satisfyingly on a gorgeous Marlboro Red.

I was pleasantly surprised about how few withdrawal symptoms I had. At the time I didn't know that most withdrawal symptoms are caused by Nitch's propaganda, not by his whingeing. In the Arctic there was absolutely no option of smoking. Usually when you quit Nitch comes up with endless excuses and justifications to make you start again and it is this constant commentary about whether you should/shouldn't smoke that is so stressful and exhausting. But if there is no possibility of smoking, then Nitch falls silent. He can't influence your decisions because there aren't any to be made.

Nevertheless I was eagerly anticipating the pleasures of the first post-trip cigarette. In fact my first truly powerful craving to smoke began as soon as the possibility of smoking became a reality. We had planned to be back in civilisation by noon, plenty of time before the shops shut. But the boat was delayed and we didn't get back until nightfall. This was still a very remote settlement and nothing was open. Suddenly, having coped perfectly well with not smoking for nine weeks, I found the prospect of one more night without cigarettes unbearable.

Another group of mountaineers was camped nearby so I asked them for a cigarette and, joy of joys, they had plenty. I lit up, inhaled deeply and...nothing. I felt a bit sick but I was expecting that because I hadn't smoked for ages. I also expected it to taste grim, because I never really liked the taste of cigarettes, but there was something hugely wrong with the cigarette that went beyond just not tasting very nice. It wasn't satisfying.

I now realise that it wasn't satisfying because I had absolutely no nicotine in my body. So there was no *dis*-satisfaction to relieve. But at that time I was bewildered, frustrated and deeply disappointed. 'The cigarette isn't working,' I said plaintively. 'There's something wrong with it.' Of course, there was nothing wrong with the cigarette. It was just that if you have no need of nicotine then cigarettes do not satisfy.

Unfortunately I didn't know that then, and I decided the fags were stale and that I would buy a new pack the next day. Which I did. I still had this image in my mind, and many memories of 'enjoyable' and 'satisfying' cigarettes, and I didn't know they were misconceptions. After three more useless cigarettes that didn't work, I finally smoked one that felt the way they used to feel. Lucky me – I had just reincarnated Nitch and now could 'enjoy' cigarettes again. That misunderstanding cost me another year of smoking.

If you are still convinced that you smoke because you like the taste, think about what you would do if there were no brands that you liked on offer. When I was a smoker I hated menthol cigarettes. The mintiness affected the way the smoke felt on the back of my throat and didn't feel right. But if there was nothing else available, would I smoke menthols or go without? Smoke them, of course. In fact, I've been known to smoke butts out of old ashtrays rather than go without cigarettes. And on one memorable occasion, I was pacing the house, unable to leave because I was babysitting and unable to find my cigarettes because my sister had nicked them. (I'd give my sister my house, but my cigarettes? You've got to be joking.)

I was frantically searching in pockets of old coats and in the depths of handbags and to my delight I found a cigarette. So it was a bit green and damp looking but, hey, a fag is a fag. I smoked it and while I can assure you that it was not in the least tasty, it certainly satisfied. There is a big difference. Enjoyment is something extra you get from doing or having something nice. Smoking is simply the temporary relief of dissatisfaction and misery.

leisure and social smoking

Other cigarettes that people find most 'pleasurable' or enjoyable are those they smoke when they are out socially, or when they are relaxing. In these situations they are doing things that are themselves genuinely pleasurable. They may be out with friends, or at a party, or unwinding after work. One of my favourite cigarettes was the one I had as soon as I got home from work. I had a whole ritual surrounding this precious cigarette. I would change into comfortable clothes, make a cup of tea, put on some relaxing music, then sit on the sofa, put my feet up and light up.

If you pair something irrelevant with something nice over and over again, the thing that you have paired with the pleasure becomes pleasurable in itself. In the situation I have just described, all the things I was doing were genuinely pleasurable and relaxing. The cigarette became associated with these pleasures till it seemed as if it was the cigarette itself that was the most important thing. If you always smoke in situations when you are relaxing, drinking, socialising or unwinding, then the cigarette becomes associated with those pleasures, and you feel that the cigarette is a crucial part of them. When you first quit, these situations feel odd, as if there is something missing. What the research has shown, however, is that if you break the link, the conditioning fades. You will therefore find that you enjoy the genuine pleasures of those situations as much as you ever did. (We'll look at this concept in more detail in the next chapter.)

enhancing enjoyment of other activities

Another reason why the belief that smoking makes good times even better is to do with Nitch, and how he behaves if you do not smoke. Smokers often find that they cannot enjoy situations when they are not smoking. No matter how good their holiday is, it just would not be enjoyable without smoking.

So isn't that good evidence of the value of cigarettes? They make good times even better? No! This is another misconception. Another cost in disguise. People don't enjoy things more if they can smoke – but they certainly enjoy them less if they can't. *This is not the same thing!* If you are smoking, Nitch will allow you to enjoy the rest of your holiday. But he won't add anything to it.

Smoking is irrelevant when you are doing it. It's just there, like part of the furniture. But when you can't smoke, or if it is difficult to smoke, Nitch will make an awful fuss and prevent you from enjoying anything, or will insist that you suffer significant inconvenience to feed

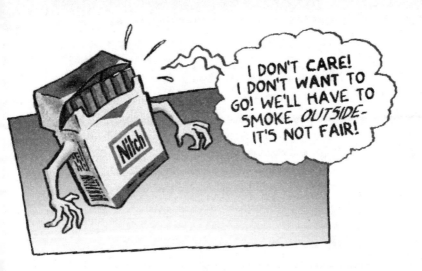

him. I ski every year and usually a group of friends and I stay in a hosted chalet. Since there are usually more non-smokers than smokers among the other guests, smoking is not permitted in the chalet. This year there was only one smoker who had to stand outside in the freezing cold by himself every time Nitch needed feeding. So in the evenings we would all be sitting around by the lovely log fire, chatting, drinking red wine and playing cards, while he was shivering outside getting his nicotine fix. Smoking didn't add anything at all to his holiday. It just got in the way. (Isn't it funny how smokers in those sorts of situations will say, 'I like the fresh air' but when they quit they never feel the urge to experience sub-zero 'fresh air' in the middle of the night again?) How much nicer it is not to have to think about Nitch, or worry about him, or pander to his endless demands.

In one of my groups a woman told me that her daughter had recently got married. As she sat in church watching her daughter's wedding ceremony, all she was thinking was, 'I hope they hurry up, because I really want a cigarette.' That was a perfect (though tragic) example of how cigarettes get in the way of enjoyment and destroy special occasions while adding absolutely nothing of value at all. And this is not a unique occurrence – quitting adviser Allen Carr admits to having had the same experience at his own daughter's wedding before he gave up.

concentration

'Okay, okay, maybe cigarettes are stressful and it's a pain to have to smoke all the time. But if I didn't smoke, I just couldn't function properly. I need to smoke to keep me focused at work.'

People will often say that smoking helps them concentrate. It keeps them sharp. It adds an edge of creativity. If you are stuck at work, what better way to unstick yourself than to have a fag. Afterwards solutions present themselves and you can think more clearly.

Nonsense! This is just another cost cunningly disguised as a benefit.

In the same way that cigarettes make you stressed while pretending they are helping you feel less stressed, cigarettes destroy your ability to concentrate while pretending to improve it. Imagine trying to concentrate on your job with a tantrumming toddler demanding Smarties from you. Nitch operates the same way. And he is tremendously distracting. When he wants feeding (which is most of the time) he will not let it rest. He cannot take no for an answer. And he won't rest till you give in and feed him. Just like the toddler he then pipes down, so you can heave a sigh of relief and get on with some work…till next time!

But again, instead of blaming smoking for creating such an endless distraction, you assume that the cigarette actually gives your concentration a boost. This is another example of Nitch's power over you. He manages to distract you and impair your concentration day in and day out while at the same time making you believe that cigarettes (his lifeline) are wonderfully helpful to you.

addiction

'Okay, so maybe all I'm doing is feeding an addiction. Knowing that doesn't make it any easier to stop. After all, beating addiction is incredibly difficult. And smoking is one of the hardest of them all.'

It is certainly true that nicotine is highly addictive. But this does not mean that you can't escape. Addiction is poorly understood and there are many misconceptions about addicts, such as 'once an addict always an addict'. These misconceptions developed because of the great difficulty some people have in giving up smoking. Other evidence shows that some people who do stop smoking still crave cigarettes. You may meet people who tell you that they quit ten years ago and still could 'murder a fag'. Other people will tell you that despite long-term success in quitting, they still feel as if they are addicts: 'If I had one I'd go straight back to twenty a day.'

You yourself may have quit for months and years before, but nonetheless felt drawn to smoking and had to use constant willpower to stay off cigarettes.

Despite all this, it is still untrue to say that people cannot be totally free. It is certainly true that some people quit and continue to crave cigarettes long after all nicotine has disappeared from their bodies. However, research into ex-smokers also shows that many of them do not continue to crave. Many look back on their smoking with bafflement – they remember how important cigarettes seemed at the time, but they can't for the life of them figure out why! They no longer relate to smoking. Often they find the smell offensive and they have no idea what on earth made them do it for so long. These are not people who are constantly having to exert willpower. They are truly free from smoking and cigarettes are now completely unimportant in their lives.

Okay, you might say, all that shows is that some people are lucky enough not to have addictive personalities. But actually the research is more complicated and interesting than that: the same smoker can sometimes quit and never miss cigarettes afterwards, and yet sometimes quit and find themselves suffering terrible cravings.

So how come they started smoking again if they didn't miss smoking at all? Good point – I'm glad you're paying attention! The answer is simply that there are many pitfalls that trap unwary non-smokers or ex-smokers. People who are totally free can still get hooked again. There is a whole chapter later on devoted to the important issue of preventing a relapse once you have managed to get yourself free. At the moment, all you need to know is that you can quit and be totally free (i.e. you do not miss cigarettes at all) or you can quit and still not be free (i.e. you continue to miss cigarettes and crave them). And the same smoker can experience both types of quitting. The message therefore is that there is nothing inherent in a person's brain, soul or personality that makes it impossible to quit and be free. Everyone can be free, including you.

Let's take a closer look at addiction and its different definitions. People claim to be addicted to almost anything – chocolate or sex for example. One definition of addiction is that there is a change in your body when you withdraw from a substance. Heroin is a good example of that. Smoking is also an example of a substance that changes the way you feel when it leaves your system. The problem with smoking is that the nature of the withdrawal is far from understood and it varies dramatically from person to person and even in the same person on different occasions. Studies of withdrawal show that the actual physical changes in people's bodies are not what they complain about. Indeed, many people don't even notice these physical changes. What people do complain about are emotional states like grouchiness or irritability.

People can experience a similar sort of grouchiness or irritability when they go without substances that are not generally addictive, as compulsive gamblers do, for example. So part of withdrawal is psychological.

Some people use a descriptive definition of addiction. They simply describe behaviours and feelings that people have towards certain substances to decide if a person is addicted to a particular substance or not. The central feature of any addiction is so-called compulsive use. This means that people will go to great lengths to obtain the substance, and that they experience distress without it. The label addiction does not explain why a person has compulsive use. It simply describes what people do and feel.

This definition of addiction fits smokers, who make great efforts to get cigarettes and feel stressed, anxious or downright panicky without them. But it is not an explanation of smoking. The questions you need to ask yourself are:

- *Why* do I have a compulsive need to smoke?
- *Why* will I go to such ridiculous lengths to get a cigarette and
- *Why* am I so miserable without my fags?

The answer can again be found in our little villain, Nitch. Nitch can physically make you feel stressed all the time by inducing withdrawal symptoms after each cigarette. As we have seen, these lead to anxiety which we reduce by smoking again.

But this happens in our unconscious and we are completely unaware of it. So we need to find another reason. Which brings us onto Nitch's second weapon, propaganda, which makes us believe that we need cigarettes in order to be relaxed or confident, sociable, good at our job – simply to function at our best. It is not a physical state but an emotional one.

These beliefs make quitting much harder. Added to the real anxiety of nicotine withdrawal, you have the emotional turmoil of imagining life without your precious cigarettes.

A woman in one of my groups recently started using the drug bupropion (Zyban) to help her quit (more on this later). She was to take one tablet a day for six days while continuing to smoke. From day seven, still smoking, she was to take two tablets a day. On day eleven she was to quit smoking. Her 'withdrawal symptoms' began on day nine – while she was still smoking. By the end of day ten they were so bad that she didn't dare take her evening tablet. She knew that she was meant to stop the following day, and this filled her with so much panic that she stopped using the drugs altogether and abandoned the quit attempt before it even began.

Her misery was not about withdrawal. It was about dread and panic at the *thought* of withdrawal.

Another person in the group returned for his follow-up and was deeply unhappy because he had failed to stop.

'I just couldn't do it,' he said.

'What went wrong?' I asked. 'What made it so difficult to stop?'

'The withdrawal symptoms,' he replied.

'At what point did you give in to the withdrawal symptoms and smoke?'

'As soon as I woke up.'

This man went on to describe how terrible he felt as soon as he woke up, and how desperately he was craving cigarettes. These awful feelings had nothing at all to do with physical withdrawal symptoms. If he hadn't been quitting he would have felt fine on waking, even though he would have been experiencing exactly the same amount of physical withdrawal.

habit

Smokers tend to smoke at the same times and in the same places. When you quit it feels harder to enjoy those situations. Something feels missing. Smoking just seems to complete those situations. This is an important point that needs to be addressed – because *habit* is the third corner of our smoking triangle. Read on...

chapter summary

• Cigarettes appear to relax you, because they take away the anxiety they cause – for a while.

• Cigarettes appear satisfying because they create dissatisfaction then take it away again – for a while.

• Cigarettes appear to help you enjoy yourself because Nitch makes you miserable if you don't feed him.

• Cigarettes appear to help you concentrate because they distract you, then restore your concentration – for a while.

• Seeing through Nitch's propaganda is an important part of quitting.

○ ○

Worksheet 1

Understand what can go wrong in quit attempts if you haven't understood Nitch's dirty tricks. Read the following account by a man talking about his quit attempt.

I tried to quit last week but it was a bad time at work. On quit date I was having a really difficult day. My boss was getting at me and I was under a lot of pressure. I really needed to focus and concentrate on this big project and smoking helps me with that. So I decided after a terrible morning to give up the quit attempt till the weekend when I was not under so much pressure.

Saturday morning was my next attempt. It was going okay till about ten o'clock when my grandchildren came over. I love them dearly but they are a real handful and frankly their behaviour was pretty terrible. Well, I couldn't cope with them at all. They were really winding me up and I could feel that I would lose my temper with them. So I went and bought a packet and they helped me to cope with the kids. Actually smoking really does stop me being so irritable. I deal with everything much better when I can have a smoke, so I am worried about the impact quitting will have on my family.

Anyway, I'd blown it for Saturday so I thought I'd try Sunday. It was fine till the afternoon when I went to play golf with some friends. They all smoke and were pretty dismissive of my attempt to quit, telling me what a waste of time that was, and warning me of the misery ahead. So that didn't help much. After the game we were in the clubhouse having a beer, and they offered me a cigarette. Well, I couldn't relax and have a good time without one and after a long and difficult week at work I felt I deserved to be able to unwind. I started thinking that I'd much rather be relaxed and happy even if that meant damaging my health. Health is important, of course, but it's not everything. I don't want to be a miserable old sod for the rest of my days. I felt tired of punishing myself and thought I needed and deserved to be able to relax with my friends. Smoking helps me do that. So I had a few.

All in all, when I think back on how the week has gone, I reckon that despite the costs and risks, I'd rather just keep smoking for the moment. Maybe when I retire next year I'll give it another go.

○ ○ ○ ○ ○ ○ ○ ○ ○ ○ ○ ○ ○ ○ ○ ○ ○ ○ ○

Can you identify any thinking errors in this account?
Which ones?
Is he falling for the 'fundamental misconception'?
Re-read Chapters 4 and 5 if necessary.
The following page discusses some of the errors he is making. Try
to identify some of them yourself before you read on.

Let's look at the account again:

I tried to quit last week but it was a bad time at work. On quit date I was
having a really difficult day. My boss was getting at me and I was under a lot
of pressure. *I really needed to focus and concentrate on this big project and smoking
helps me with that.*

This is an example of the fundamental misconception. The belief
is that smoking helps concentration. The smoker believes that the
pressure of work is to blame for the problems in concentrating,
and the cigarette helps him to sharpen up. In reality the drop in
nicotine is to blame for the problems in concentrating and having
a cigarette relieves this distraction.

So I decided after a terrible morning to give up the quit attempt till the
weekend when I was not under so much pressure.

Saturday morning was my next attempt. It was going okay till about ten
o'clock when my grandchildren came over. I love them dearly but they are a
real handful and frankly their behaviour was pretty terrible. *Well, I couldn't cope
with them at all. They were really winding me up and I could feel that I would lose
my temper with them. So I went and bought a packet and they helped me to cope with
the kids. Actually smoking really does stop me being so irritable.*

Here again the smoker is being tricked by the fundamental
misconception. He is blaming his grandchildren for the increase in
his irritability. They are winding him up. However, once he has
had a smoke, the same behaviours no longer wind him up. Why

not? Because it wasn't them at all that were winding him up. Rather, the drop in nicotine levels was causing irritability, and the cigarette relieved that irritability. Nitch was annoying him, not his grandchildren. The man is, however, blaming the children instead of Nitch for his tension. So he believes cigarettes are actually helpful to him rather than being the cause of his problems.

I deal with everything much better when I can have a smoke, so I am worried about the impact quitting will have on my family.

The fundamental misconception described above leads him to a general conclusion about the impact of smoking on his relationships. This is an example of over-generalisation. The generalisation is that smoking helps. In reality, smoking makes him stressed and irritable. The belief that smoking helps people with irritability is a common excuse for carrying on smoking. Parents say they deal with their children better after a smoke. However, this is simply due to the fact that being a nicotine addict makes you tense and irritable. A cigarette temporarily relieves that problem.

Anyway, I'd blown it for Saturday so I thought I'd try Sunday. It was fine till the afternoon when I went to play golf with some friends. *They all smoke and were pretty dismissive of my attempt to quit, telling me what a waste of time that was, and warning me of the misery ahead.*

This is an example of sabotage, common among smokers whose friends/family are quitting. This is further discussed later in the book.

So that didn't help much. After the game we were in the clubhouse having a beer, and they offered me a cigarette. *Well, I couldn't relax and have a good time without one.*

This is another example of the fundamental misconception. The man believes that smoking is pleasurable and relaxing. In reality, if you are a nicotine addict, it is not possible to be totally relaxed without a cigarette because nicotine withdrawal is stressful. The man is unable to

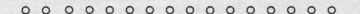

relax because he is experiencing nicotine withdrawal. Smoking temporarily removes the barrier to relaxation. Smoking because you cannot relax unless you are smoking is a very different thing from smoking because smoking is relaxing. The latter is the fundamental misconception which implies a genuine beneficial effect of smoking – pleasure and relaxation. The former, on the other hand, is similar to a person with fleas! Unless you relieve the itching, you will not have a good time. But the flea bites are not actually helping you, even though scratching them feels nice. Looking at it like that shows how difficult it is ever to relax if you are a smoker.

I started thinking that I'd much rather be relaxed and happy even if that meant damaging my health. Health is important, of course, but it's not everything. I don't want to be a miserable old sod for the rest of my days. I felt tired of punishing myself and thought I needed and deserved to be able to relax with my friends.

Again, the specific fundamental misconception has led to a general belief on the importance of smoking in this man's life.

Smoking helps me do that. So I had a few.

All in all, when I think back on how the week has gone, I reckon that despite the costs and risks, I'd rather just keep smoking for the moment. Maybe when I retire next year I'll give it another go.

This man's unhappy experiences of quitting have led him to a decision to continue smoking. However, his conclusions are based on distorted thinking. In order to quit, he needs to change his perceptions of his experiences of smoking. That is the aim of this book.

○ ○ ○ ○ ○ ○ ○ ○ ○ ○ ○ ○ ○ ○ ○ ○ ○ ○ ○

Worksheet 2: costs in disguise

Finish each of these sentences from the choices presented below.

NOT ENJOYMENT BUT _____

NOT IMPROVED CONCENTRATION BUT _____

NOT RELAXATION BUT _____

NOT PLEASURE BUT_____

NOT FREE CHOICE BUT_____

Choose from the following:

- distraction then partial relief
- addiction
- conditioning
- inability to have fun without smoking
- stress then partial relief of stress

Now add some of your own:

NOT_____ BUT_____

NOT_____ BUT_____

NOT_____ BUT_____

NOT_____ BUT_____

Habit

Most smokers smoke at certain times and places throughout the day. They will automatically light up in certain situations, without necessarily even being aware of it. When people quit, they often find that they are coping okay when they are in unfamiliar places, or places where they rarely smoked, but that as soon as they get to a 'smoking situation' the cravings suddenly intensify. Again this is evidence that withdrawal symptoms are not just physical. Your nicotine levels have not plummeted because you have walked into a pub. Some people say smoking is 'just a habit' because they notice that they can stop for long periods in some situations but light up automatically in others. Breaking the habit seems very difficult, and people often worry that they will never enjoy many of the things they used to enjoy, because cigarettes were so strongly associated with them.

Cravings can also be triggered when people see or smell cigarettes, for example catching sight of a cigarette kiosk at the supermarket or walking past the Duty Free Shop at an airport. This places people at risk of buying cigarettes on impulse. But why should the sight of cigarettes or certain places trigger cravings in someone who generally feels fine without their cigarettes? To overcome these potential problems, we need to understand why cravings are triggered. What we call 'habit' is called **conditioning** in psychology.

Many years ago a scientist named Pavlov described **classical conditioning**. What he did was to notice that dogs tended to produce saliva when they were presented with food. This salivation was called the **unconditioned response**, meaning that it was a natural response to the smell and sight of food.

What Pavlov did next was to ring a bell whenever he fed the dogs. This meant that the dogs salivated whenever they saw or smelled food, but they also salivated when they heard a bell. The bell was irrelevant, but the dogs salivated when they heard it, because they always heard it at the same time as they were given food.

Next Pavlov rang the bell, *without* offering the dogs any food. The dogs began to salivate as soon as they heard the bell. This was called the **conditioned response**. There is no reason why a dog should salivate when it hears a bell, but in this instance the dogs had learned to associate the bell with food.

So how does this relate to smoking? Well, conditioning is now clearly understood as the process by which something irrelevant takes on meaning by being paired with something that is meaningful, and this has several implications for smoking.

The taste, smell and sensations of smoking are irrelevant. You smoke for the nicotine because the nicotine provides relief. But every time you experience satisfaction and relief of nicotine withdrawal, lots of other stimuli are present at the same time. The handling of the cigarettes, the taste and smell, the sensation of smoke entering your lungs and the flicking of the ash are all present every time you get relief from nicotine withdrawal. So you start to associate other aspects of smoking with the relief. You therefore start to believe that these things on their own are important. They are not. You have just been programmed or conditioned to see them as important.

Key Concept

Smokers have been conditioned to think of the taste and sensation of smoking as satisfying because they associate these things with relief of nicotine withdrawal.

Key Concept

We become conditioned to see smoking as pleasurable and relaxing if we always smoke in pleasurable and relaxing situations.

When people quit, they miss all these associated bits. They miss the feel of cigarettes in their hand and the ritual of buying the packets from the newsagent. Walking past the rows of shiny packs causes a pang of loss for smokers when they first quit.

In addition, when you smoke in the same situations every day, the cigarettes become associated with those situations. They are often relaxing, or are paired with other pleasant things. For example, smoking your first cigarette of the day with a cup of coffee, smoking during work breaks, coming home from work and sitting down with a cup of tea and a cigarette, smoking in a pub, smoking when a particular friend comes round, smoking while drinking wine or beer.

These situations themselves are pleasant and relaxing. The cigarette initially is irrelevant. But if you smoke whenever you are in particular situations, you gradually start to associate those pleasant feelings with the smoking. This is a conditioned response. Smoking is not the relaxing bit about coming home from work, putting your feet up and having a cup of tea, but it becomes associated with those things and takes on their qualities.

So just like the dog salivating over something irrelevant (a bell) because it is associated with something relevant (food), you relax or feel good over something irrelevant (a cigarette) because it is associated with something relevant (relaxation, leisure, sociability).

Once this conditioned response has developed, you will find that those situations trigger thoughts of smoking. If you are trying to quit, those situations may trigger cravings.

So how do you escape from this angle of the Smoking Triangle? Well, Pavlov took his experiments a little further. What he found was that when you broke the link between the stimulus (the bell) and the things it was associated with (the food), the dogs gradually stopped associating the bell with food. The bell lost its power. This process was called **extinction**.

What this means for smoking is that when you stop smoking, all those situations where you usually smoked feel weird at first. When you quit you will obviously still continue to see and smell cigarettes, and in situations where you have always smoked in the past, you will feel you are missing out, because you will still have some positive associations. But as long as you don't smoke, the association between the sight and smell of a cigarette and relief or satisfaction will fade away. In addition, the association between pleasure, sociability, relaxation and friendship will also fade away. So the link between smoking and those situations will gradually be extinguished. Once this has happened, you will be able to enjoy the genuinely relaxing aspects to life as much as ever before, without feeling you are missing out on anything. In fact you will be able to enjoy them more than ever before because you won't have the hassle of dealing with Nitch whenever you are out. You will never again experience the awful and irritating twitchiness that smokers suffer so often.

The only exception to this rule is when your beliefs about smoking are still distorted. If you firmly believe that there is something wonderful about handling a cigarette, that belief will lead you to crave cigarettes even long after the conditioned response has broken down. People who fall into this trap have a strong memory of how satisfying cigarettes were, and they keep this memory alive and well. These false memories make quitting endless – you are free of nicotine but Nitch is still in your head nagging you to smoke. Many people in this situation eventually get fed up of never feeling free of smoking and are at very high risk of relapse. That is why you need to tackle *all three angles* of the Smoking Triangle to be completely free.

One crucial part of Pavlov's work was to notice what happened if you broke the link between the bell and the food most of the time, but paired the two together occasionally. This is the equivalent of not smoking most of the time, but having the odd cigarette in certain situations. Pavlov found that if you sometimes paired two things together, then extinction *did not take place*. If the food was occasionally still paired with a bell, the dogs would continue to get very excited and drool when they heard a bell.

So in order to conquer this habit you need to break the links completely. If you quit totally, then the links disappear and your problems will be over. If you 'cheat' occasionally, then the links will not disappear: you will still 'drool' and will never be completely free.

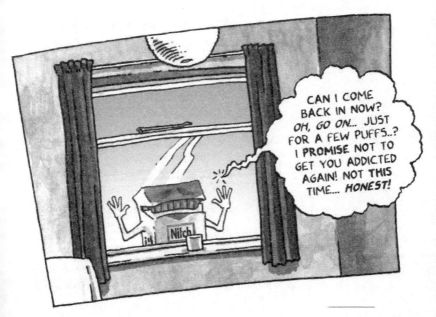

You will still associate smoking with pleasure and relaxation long after you have 'quit'. This is another reason why social smoking is very difficult to sustain and miserable even if you can do it. Social smokers never break free of the third angle. In fact they never truly break free of any of the angles: they are still addicted to nicotine (or they become regularly re-addicted if they smoke very occasionally); they still hold positive beliefs about smoking (or why would they bother with it at all); and they still have a conditioned response. Do not make life harder for yourself! Quitting must mean quitting completely.

Key Concept

If you stop smoking the conditioning vanishes. If you smoke occasionally it doesn't.

To overcome the conditioned response all you need to do is stop pairing cigarettes with any pleasurable situation. This will happen automatically if you quit. Simply being aware of what is happening when cravings are triggered can really help. However, if you want to reduce the cravings you experience, then you can take some practical steps to limit the conditioned response:

tips to help you break the conditioned response

- Vary your routines. Move furniture round your living room. Change the order in which you do things. These all help to break the link between specific situations and smoking. This might seem strange, but even simple changes like these make a big difference.

• Do not confuse the genuinely pleasurable with the conditioned response. If something is pleasurable in its own right, do it anyway. You may not enjoy it at first because it reminds you that you are not smoking, but if you persist, then the genuine pleasures of the activity come back, while the link with smoking disappears.

• Be patient. You have smoked for a long time. It may take a while before not smoking feels comfortable and familiar.

• Don't panic if cravings are unexpectedly triggered a long time after quitting. This can and will happen occasionally. If there are certain situations in which you always used to smoke, but you have not revisited them for a long time, the desire to smoke may be triggered the first time you are in that situation again. This happened to me. I used to live in London and got the tube home from work every day. As I left the station I would light up and smoke my first post-work cigarette while I walked the rest of the way home. I then moved out of London, and many years later stopped smoking. Two years after that, I returned to London to visit friends. I had not been back to that part of the city since quitting smoking. I got out at my old tube station, started walking down the same street and automatically reached into my jacket pocket for my cigarettes! Fortunately I did not panic. I realised that the link between this street and smoking had not been extinguished because I had not been back, and that the old behaviour was being triggered – the way a smell can send you back in time. I did not smoke, and the next time I walked down the street the link was no longer there.

• Remember that a craving is a *feeling* not a *command*. Accept it. It won't last long and as long as you don't smoke, it will eventually disappear for ever.

chapter summary

- If things are paired together often enough they become strongly associated with each other. This is called conditioning.

- We are conditioned to see things like taste, flicking ash, seeing packets in a shop, pulling out the silver foil and handling a cigarette as satisfying because they all become associated with relief of nicotine withdrawal.

- We are also conditioned to see cigarettes as relaxing because we smoke in relaxing and sociable places.

- If you break the link between smoking and these places, the conditioned response disappears.

- If you occasionally smoke the link remains.

- This means that occasional smoking actually makes quitting harder.

Killing Nitch: Understanding Withdrawal

8

We have learnt about the three angles of the Smoking Triangle: physical addiction, psychological dependence and habit. To summarise:

angle 1: addiction

If you smoke you will quickly start to experience nicotine withdrawal. This will cause anxiety which is interpreted by your subconscious mind as danger. You will feel compelled to reduce this anxiety by doing whatever worked best last time – which will always be smoking. When you smoke your anxiety will drop and so smoking is reinforced. You have no idea that this is happening to you. This is Nitch's first weapon – anxiety. Nitch feeds on nicotine and he makes you anxious when nicotine is running low.

The process is a vicious circle:

- The more addicted you get, the more anxiety you have.
- The more anxiety you have, the more relief you experience when you smoke. The more relief you experience when you smoke, the more powerful the drive to reduce anxiety by smoking becomes.
- The more powerful the drive to reduce anxiety by smoking becomes, the more you smoke.
- The more you smoke, the more addicted you get.

angle 2: psychological dependence

You have no idea what is happening in angle 1. You don't understand the drive to smoke, so you find it hard to explain your smoking. But you know you smoke and that smoking is deadly. So you enter a state of cognitive dissonance.

This is psychologically very uncomfortable, so you search for an alternative explanation for your smoking, while at the same time downplaying your fears of smoking. This gives rise to psychological dependence. This is Nitch's second weapon – propaganda. Nitch needs you to feed him, so he fills your head with rubbish about smoking. You listen to this nonsense because you are actively looking for an explanation for your smoking.

This is another vicious circle:

- The more you smoke, the more the costs of smoking mount up.
- The more the costs of smoking mount up, the more cognitive dissonance you experience.
- The more cognitive dissonance you experience, the more you need to downplay risks and elevate benefits.
- The more you downplay risks and elevate benefits, the more you smoke.

angle 3: habit

You tend to smoke in the same places and at the same times. This means that you start to associate smoking with the genuine pleasures or benefits of those times, such as a meal out or a work break. This process is called conditioning (or habit) and triggers powerful desires to smoke in certain places. These pleasure associations make psychological dependence more powerful because smoking itself will start to take on the qualities inherent in those situations. Habit is a major reason why people start smoking again in 'high-risk situations'; they may be fine in most situations but can still experience cravings if they go somewhere they always used to smoke. If you understand what is happening it is much easier to ride out the craving and break the links between high-risk situations and smoking.

killing Nitch:
the two types of withdrawal

To overcome nicotine addiction, you need to cut off Nitch's nicotine supply – and kill him! So you have to go through nicotine withdrawal.

Nicotine withdrawal symptoms are feelings of edginess, tension, irritability or anxiety. Think back to when you last really needed a cigarette. Well, that edgy feeling is nicotine withdrawal. It is quite mild on its own, which is why most people can spend twelve hours on a long-haul flight and cope perfectly well without smoking.

The vagueness and mildness of the symptoms is, ironically, what makes smoking so difficult to understand. There are no euphoric effects that you have to give up, and there are no powerful physical withdrawal symptoms to overcome. People are aware that they feel powerfully driven to smoke, but they don't know why, and the strength of the compulsion seems totally out of proportion to what cigarettes offer in return.

This leads smokers to search for alternative explanations for their habit, so the second process that occurs for all addicts is psychological dependence. Addicts come to believe that they need their drug and that they cannot cope without it. Together these two processes form a formidable barrier to quitting. The relative importance of each is different for all drugs, but thoughts, beliefs and attitudes are crucial in all addictions. Even an addiction like heroin which looks mostly physical is in fact largely psychological. This is why people go back to the drug even after detox. Such people are no longer physically dependent, but they still feel they need the drug. The power of psychological processes is even more apparent for those addictions that are not physical at all, such as to food, sex, work or gambling. Compulsive gamblers, for example, are not physically dependent, but they still experience intense physical symptoms when deprived of their 'fix'.

'Withdrawal' symptoms are in fact a combination of **physical withdrawal**, caused by reductions in levels of nicotine in the bloodstream, and **psychological withdrawal**, caused by your beliefs and attitudes about smoking. This leads to lots of confusion about nicotine withdrawal. All smokers experience it, but no one experiences it in exactly the same way as anyone else. Physical withdrawal involves your body ridding itself of the nicotine on which it has become dependent. This process kills Nitch, and his death throes can be felt by the person he lives in. Psychological withdrawal is a powerful process caused by feelings of loss, fear, deprivation, misery and stress. This is where Nitch's propaganda machine is at its most effective.

Key Concept

Nicotine withdrawal is a combination of physical withdrawal and psychological withdrawal.

Nitch's running commentary, aimed at keeping you smoking, makes quitting seem overwhelmingly difficult and leaves smokers feeling anxious and miserable at the thought of giving up. It is important to remember that at this stage these thoughts are just that – *thoughts*. They have no external reality. They are not real experiences.

Key Concept

Thoughts are just thoughts.
They do not have external reality.

It is the thoughts themselves that give rise to anxiety and misery. It is not quitting that does this, since the anxiety and misery develop before you even quit. The way you think is making you feel terrible. If you change the way you think, you will also change how you feel and how you experience quitting.

To illustrate how thinking affects how you experience quitting, think about times when smoking is absolutely impossible. If there is no possibility of smoking, then Nitch falls silent. He can't influence your decisions because there aren't any to be made. Remember my account of the trip to the Arctic. I went from thirty a day to zero overnight. And the withdrawal symptoms I experienced were nothing like as bad as I had expected. Considering the terrible symptoms I had had when I was trying to quit in the past, this didn't make much sense at the time. Now I realise that in the Arctic all I experienced was physical withdrawal, and that the misery I went through in other attempts to give up was mostly Nitch driving me round the bend with his endless doom and gloom about the tragedy of a smoke-free life. If you no longer believe in Nitch's propaganda, or if you are in a place where smoking is totally impossible, then the second aspect of withdrawal is not experienced.

If people believe they want and need cigarettes, these beliefs will lead to fear and therefore present a barrier to quitting. This fear and misery confirm your belief that you need to smoke, and a vicious circle develops. The more miserable you feel, the more you believe that you cannot live without cigarettes, and the more you believe that you cannot live without cigarettes, the more misery and fear you feel.

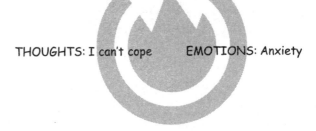

THOUGHTS: I can't cope   EMOTIONS: Anxiety

In this way, the misery and fear become a self-fulfilling prophecy, and people do feel wretched and miserable if they stop smoking. If you change your thinking, then you will have a different experience of quitting, even though the external reality is the same.

Key Concept

> **Changing the way you think, changes the way you feel.**

Most people know that heroin is addictive and that if you quit you go 'cold turkey'. This is viewed by heroin users and non-users alike as a terrible ordeal. When servicemen were in Vietnam many thousands of them began to use heroin regularly to numb themselves from the horrors of war. Naturally they all got addicted and it was widely believed that this addiction was going to be a serious problem when the soldiers returned home. Against all expectations, most of the men gave up heroin easily and permanently as soon as they returned. This can be explained in terms of the two types of withdrawal. The men knew perfectly well why they were using heroin in Vietnam. They did not feel stupid about it as they saw it as a necessary shield against the horror they were regularly subjected to. Because they had genuine reasons for using heroin they were not susceptible to the sort of Nitch-driven justifications that smokers use. So when they got home the only problem was the physical withdrawal from heroin and, although this is unpleasant, on its own it is manageable.

Similarly, most people do not become addicted to pain relief if they use it to relieve pain, even if they are using drugs that are addictive when used recreationally or for other reasons. The difficulty in curing addiction lies in the beliefs about drugs that addicts hold. Rid yourself of these beliefs and killing Nitch becomes no more than a few days of mild stress and perhaps sleeplessness.

Think about your own experiences of withdrawal. Most smokers start craving cigarettes soon after stubbing out their last one on a quit attempt. This is before Nitch has even begun to whimper. Conversely, many smokers can go for hours and hours without smoking. If your mental state is right for quitting, withdrawal is not a problem.

Key Concept

Most withdrawal symptoms are psychological.

So what does this mean for quitting? Well, it means you have to free yourself from *both* processes. You need to overcome the physical dependence by cutting off the supply of nicotine and therefore killing Nitch. And you have to change the way you think about smoking, so that you no longer remain psychologically hooked. Many quit attempts just focus on getting over the physical dependence. The problem there is that people who are physically free but psychologically hooked do not feel free. They feel deprived and miserable. They may even still experience physical cravings, which are no less real to the sufferer just because they originate in their head.

You may meet people who quit years and years ago but still crave cigarettes. This observation has led many people, including some healthcare professionals, to believe that you can never truly overcome an addiction. Instead you have to learn to live with being 'in recovery' for ever. While it is true that some people never seem to get over it, others clearly do. The important question therefore is what is the difference between ex-addicts who feel totally free, and those who still feel trapped? The answer is that the addicts who still feel trapped have not changed their internal tapes about the drug. They have only won half the war. Those who feel totally free have freed themselves from physical and psychological dependence.

Key Concept

People who quit a long time ago and still miss cigarettes only freed themselves from nicotine addiction, not from psychological dependence. They only did half the job!

Freeing yourself from physical dependence means cutting off the supply of the drug, allowing it to leave your body and allowing your body to readapt to life without the drug. There are products such as various types of Nicotine Replacement Therapy (NRT) or the drug bupropion (Zyban) that can help you.

However, freeing yourself from physical addiction is not enough on its own. You also need to free yourself from psychological dependence, and you need to overcome the habit of smoking.

The next three chapters deal with each of these in turn.

chapter summary

- Quitting smoking involves tackling all three angles of the Smoking Triangle.

- Angle 1 is nicotine addiction, which you can think of as Nitch making you anxious whenever his nicotine levels drop.

- Angle 2 is psychological dependence, which is the positive beliefs you have about smoking. This can be seen as Nitch's propaganda.

- Angle 3 is habit. Habit or conditioning refers to the way in which you have gradually come to associate smoking with pleasure, relaxation or reduced stress. Nitch will use this habitual smoking as part of his propaganda machine.

- Withdrawal is a combination of physical and psychological withdrawal.

- If you deal with all three angles of the Smoking Triangle then you will overcome both types of withdrawal.

Overcoming angle 1: nicotine addiction

To help you overcome physical addiction to nicotine, there are several products available over the counter or on prescription. The two main products available to UK smokers are Nicotine Replacement Therapies (NRT) and bupropion (Zyban). NRT works by replacing some of the nicotine you get from a cigarette, which reduces the intensity of withdrawal symptoms and cravings. Bupropion, which is only available on prescription, does not contain any nicotine and works directly on brain pathways that are affected by addictive processes.

nicotine replacement therapy (NRT)

Smoking kills approximately half of all smokers. However, it is not the nicotine in cigarettes that does the most damage. Nicotine is not in itself a primary cause of smoking-related disease or death (though it does have some harmful effects). The devastation of smoking is caused by the 'tar', a black, sticky substance containing over 4,000 chemicals which include many known cancer-causing agents and poisons. Nicotine is what makes smoking addictive, but it is the tar that destroys your health and kills you. NRT aims to replace the nicotine you get from smoking in different, far safer ways.

> ### Key Concept
>
> Nicotine is safer than tar. So NRT is much safer than cigarettes.

There are many ways of using NRT. The options available in the UK are:

- skin patches
- chewing gum
- under the tongue tablets
- lozenges
- nasal sprays
- inhalers

There are various brands available, and the products come in different strengths, but they all work in the same way: they provide an alternative method of getting nicotine.

All types of NRT are available on prescription to smokers over the age of eighteen. If you are under eighteen, your doctor may agree to prescribe them for you, but you will need to discuss this with him or her. If you have health problems or are pregnant or breast-feeding, your doctor has the right to refuse to prescribe NRT on the grounds that nicotine may be harmful to your health. This sounds like sensible practice but if you are asking your GP for NRT it is safe to assume that you are smoking. You are therefore getting the nicotine anyway, plus the 4,000 other chemicals. The National Institute for Health and Clinical Excellence (NICE) is a recognised and respected authority on all clinical matters. NICE supports the use of NRT in pregnancy.

If you want NRT then arrange to see your GP for a discussion about your health and medical history. You can take along the table shown on the next page to help you have a frank and informed discussion about the risks and benefits of using NRT in pregnancy. Alternatively, you could try an over-the-counter product, or ask to see another GP.

Nearly a hundred trials have been conducted to look at the effectiveness of NRT and they clearly show that NRT can help

NRT prescribing in pregnancy or illness: NICE guidelines

Nicotine is not the primary cause of death or morbidity. Rather it is the 4000 chemicals in the tar that kill. NRT is therefore far safer than smoking.

Smokers are already receiving nicotine when they smoke. Moreover, plasma nicotine levels from a cigarette are many times higher than those from NRT. This is because smoking a cigarette causes nicotine to be transported arterially via the carotid arteries, whereas NRT is transported in venous blood, and plasma levels are much lower.

In recognition of these factors, the latest guidelines from the National Institute for Health and Clinical Excellence (NICE, March 2002), *recommend the use of NRT products in pregnancy, and with patients suffering serious illness.* The NICE document reads: 'Smokers with certain conditions...are advised only to use NRT after careful consideration of risks and benefits and after discussion with a health care professional.' Similar advice applies to women who are pregnant or breast-feeding. *When giving such advice to people in these groups who have been unable to quit smoking without using a cessation aid, health care professionals should take into account the significant harm associated with continuing to smoke and that it can be expected that NRT will deliver less nicotine and none of the other potentially disease-causing agents that would be obtained from cigarettes.'*

people to stop smoking. While it is true that some trials are funded by drug manufacturers who have to prove that their drug is effective in order to be allowed to sell it, there is an extremely strict system of checks and balances in scientific research which ensures that, no matter who the funder is, the studies are impartial and tightly controlled. Many NRT trials have been conducted by independent researchers with no vested interest. They also show that NRT works.

In these trials one group of participants received NRT while another group was given a fake version or placebo. The results showed that people on NRT were twice as likely to quit smoking as those on the placebo (and there could be no psychological advantage as no-one knew who was getting the real NRT). However, using NRT does not feel the same as smoking. NRT does not produce the same effects as a cigarette, and anyone who expects it to resemble smoking will be disappointed. NRT is not a cigarette substitute.

Key Concept

NRT is extremely well researched. The evidence shows that it doubles your chance of quitting success.

Which product you choose is a matter of personal preference. They all work in the same way in that they replace the nicotine you currently get from cigarettes, which reduces physical withdrawal symptoms and cravings. Studies show that they all work equally well.

It is important that you choose the correct strength (see below) and your doctor or pharmacist can help you with that. Do not try to make do with less than you need. It will not make coming off the NRT any easier and may mean you fail to stop smoking. Studies suggest that using as much as you need is important in giving you the best chance of success. You are entitled to eight (or possibly twelve) weeks' supply on prescription. After that, you should either come off the NRT or start to buy the product over the counter.

You may assume that you get more nicotine from the NRT than from cigarettes if you look at how many milligrams of nicotine there are in cigarettes. But this is misleading. Smoking is an extremely efficient way of getting nicotine. The nicotine is carried in large arteries that run up to the brain. Seven seconds after having a puff, nicotine hits your brain. No form of NRT works like that, so do not try to compare NRT nicotine dosages with dosages on cigarette packets. You will always get less nicotine in your bloodstream from NRT than from cigarettes.

Side effects are rare and not serious. Some people are sensitive to the glue on the patches. Others experience irritation of the nose and eyes with the nasal sprays. Feel free to experiment with different types of NRT to see which one suits you. Some people suffer minor sleep disturbances, though this may also be caused by stopping smoking.

the products

Transdermal (skin) patches are worn for either sixteen or twenty-four hours per day. They are available in 5, 10 and 15mg strengths, or 7, 14 and 21mg strengths, depending on the brand. Some health professionals advise you to reduce the strength of the patch as your quit attempt continues (e.g. take each strength for four weeks, for a total course of twelve weeks). If you wish to do this, that is fine. The logic behind this is to make it easier to come off the patch. However, there is very little evidence that people find coming off the patch hard (though this is not true of other types of NRT). On the other hand, there is evidence that using reduced doses of NRT makes quitting less likely. If you feel confident that you can reduce the dose, then do so, as it can be powerfully motivating and make you feel that you are making progress. But if you are struggling, stay on the higher dose.

Similarly, if at the end of the course you feel you are coping fine and can come off the drug, then do so and congratulations! But if you are still struggling, take NRT for longer. Remember, it is always far far better to use NRT than to smoke.

Long-term use of any version of NRT does have its problems (more on this later) but it is better than going back to smoking.

Chewing gum is available in 2 or 4mg strengths and can be chewed for several hours at a time. Some people find the taste awful at first, but then they did not like the taste of cigarettes either. It is possible to get hooked on gum. Some people have been on it for years, and find it just as hard to give up as cigarettes. To avoid this, try to stick to the eight- or twelve-week programme.

Under-the-tongue tablets and lozenges are (obviously!) placed under the tongue and allowed to dissolve. Tablets come in 2mg strength while lozenges are available in 1, 2 and 4mg.

Nasal sprays deliver 0.5mg of nicotine per spray. These take a little while to get the hang of, and some people hate the sensation at first.

Inhalers are cigarette-shaped holders with a cartridge that contains 10mg of nicotine. You inhale the nicotine by sucking on the holder in the same way as with a cigarette. This does not mean the inhalers feel like smoking cigarettes. The aim of NRT is to replace some of the nicotine, not to replace smoking.

Nasal sprays and inhalers deliver nicotine quite quickly, so some people prefer them to the products that are taken by mouth or through the skin.

Key Concept

All forms and brands of NRT work in the same way and all are equally effective. Choose whichever you prefer.

long-term use

Nicotine in any form is an addictive drug. You can therefore get hooked on NRT just as easily as on cigarettes. Nicotine has been compulsively used in many different forms across cultures and throughout history. There is nothing special about a cigarette. Cigarettes just happen to be the way we get nicotine. If we lived in a different time or place we might instead be tobacco chewers or snuff users. Some Asian communities use paan, a paste containing nicotine which is rubbed on the gums.

If you get hooked on NRT you will at least be spared the 4,000 toxic chemicals that make cigarettes so deadly. But you will still be a nicotine addict and will still suffer the hassle and expense of living with Nitch. You will keep experiencing withdrawal symptoms and will have all the psychological dependency problems that make life as a smoker so unpleasant. You will not be free. If you ever go somewhere where your product is not available you will either need to fill your suitcases with NRT or go back to smoking. My hopes for you therefore are not merely that you switch from cigarettes to NRT but that you become free of the addiction altogether.

If being an NRT addict seems attractive to you, re-read the first few chapters, switching the word NRT for cigarette. Life as a smoker is difficult and stressful quite apart from the health consequences. Life as an NRT addict is just as difficult for the same reasons.

Key Concept

Nicotine is addictive in any form – including NRT.

If you feel at risk of developing an NRT dependence or if you have been hooked on NRT in the past, then try patches, as these have the least potential for longer-term addiction. This is not because the patch is not addictive – it is. However, addiction is much more powerful when psychological dependence begins to develop. With any form of nicotine use, you get physically hooked first. Then beliefs and attitudes about the importance of the drug begin to develop, and psychological dependence is created, as we have seen with cigarettes.

If you use chewing gum, beliefs also often develop about how great the chewing action feels and how good it tastes. With most forms of NRT you actually have to do something, such as inhale, spray or chew. With under-the-tongue NRT you experience the taste. Patches are the only form of NRT where, apart from slapping the thing on, you do nothing and feel nothing. For this reason it is harder to develop positive beliefs about the product and therefore makes it harder to develop psychological dependence.

However, these beliefs take time to develop, so you can safely use all the products for at least the eight to twelve weeks suggested. Just keep in mind that switching permanently to NRT is not the aim, and make sure that if you start 'liking' the NRT a bit too much, you come off it or switch to a patch.

Key Concept

There is little risk of getting hooked on patches. This is not true of all other types of NRT.

There are some advantages to using types of NRT that require conscious effort, because many people find it helpful actually to do something to help them get through a particularly difficult situation such as a party. In that case, slipping a lozenge under the tongue, for example, can provide the confidence needed to stay off cigarettes in high-risk circumstances.

dual use

NRT products are licensed to be used singly. In other words, only one product at a time. You will therefore probably be prescribed only one type of NRT. However, there are studies that show that using two types at a time is more effective than just one. Some people, for example, like to have a patch on all the time to give them a base-line of nicotine, but also to use a different form of NRT several times throughout the day when they feel they need a bit of a boost.

There is very little risk of overdosing on nicotine. Smokers have access to large amounts of nicotine in their cigarette packets. They manage, without advice from their pharmacists or GPs, to inhale as much nicotine as they need from each cigarette. People can smoke strong or weak cigarettes, and even if they have no idea whether a cigarette is high, medium or low in nicotine, they can still regulate the dose so that they get as much nicotine as they want. People will cadge strong roll-ups and smoke them without overdosing, even if normally they smoke ultra-mild cigarettes. So don't worry about using too much NRT. If you do want to use two types you will probably have to buy one of them over the counter, although some GPs are willing to prescribe more than one type.

how it works
(and why it might not...)

NRT works by replacing some of the nicotine you currently get from smoking. This should in turn lessen cravings and make staying off cigarettes easier. But remember, cravings are only partly physical. NRT does not stop you wanting or missing cigarettes if your internal tape is telling you cigarettes are special. NRT does not stop psychological dependence. If you are in the right frame of mind for quitting, NRT can be very helpful in reducing physical withdrawal symptoms. If you are in the wrong frame of mind, it will not work for you.

Key Concept

NRT can help you overcome physical addiction (angle 1) but it does not address psychological dependence.

bupropion

Bupropion is a prescription-only drug, made by GlaxoSmithKline, and marketed under the brand name Zyban. Bupropion is not considered suitable if you are pregnant or breast-feeding, or if you are under eighteen. Some GPs are reluctant to prescribe bupropion. If you want to try it, but your GP is unwilling, you could tell him or her that the use of bupropion is supported by the National Institute for Health and Clinical Excellence (NICE). Their guidelines read: 'NRT and bupropion are recommended for smokers who have expressed a desire to quit smoking.'

Most GPs will prescribe bupropion only if you are also willing to receive counselling and/or motivational support. This is a good idea as your chances of success are considerably higher if you have professional support along the way. There are free smoking-cessation services available worldwide (see page 217). Many of these will not specifically address psychological dependence as very few services are psychology-led or have input from clinical psychology. However, they can provide support, encouragement, advice on product use and health information.

Key Concept

**Bupropion is available only on prescription.
Talk to your GP if you want to try it.**

Bupropion works on brain pathways that are involved in addiction and withdrawal, but exactly how it works is not clear. It is nicotine-free and non-addictive, and trials have shown that it is successful in helping people stop smoking. There have been few trials comparing the effectiveness of bupropion and NRT: one study showed bupropion was more effective, but more research is needed to confirm this.

Key Concept

Unlike NRT, bupropion is not addictive.

Smokers using bupropion describe their cigarettes as tasting awful or failing to satisfy them any more. It is rather like smoking nicotine-free or ultra-low-yield cigarettes – they taste and smell like cigarettes but they just do not do the job! If cigarettes are less satisfying it then becomes easier to give them up, and many people feel that as long as they are still on the bupropion there is no point in smoking. Smokers also experience fewer withdrawal symptoms and fewer cravings.

Key Concept

**Bupropion appears to stop people gaining
satisfaction from a cigarette.**

side effects

Certain side effects are associated with bupropion and it is important that you discuss the risks with your doctor before starting treatment. The most clinically important is an increased risk of seizures. These occur in 0.1% of cases, i.e. one in a thousand patients. For this reason, bupropion will not be prescribed for you if you have a history of seizures, or if you have any of the other risk factors for a lowered seizure threshold. These risk factors include:

- prior seizure
- history of head injury
- central nervous system tumour
- taking other medications known to lower seizure threshold, including some antidepressants, antipsychotics,theophylline, systemic steroids, quinolone antibiotics and antimalarials
- excessive use of alcohol
- rapid withdrawal from alcohol or tranquillisers
- diabetes treated with hypoglycemics or insulin
- use of over-the-counter stimulants
- addiction to opiates, cocaine or stimulants
- history of anorexia or bulimia nervosa (serious eating disorders)

If you are taking another medication that reduces the seizure threshold, but would like to try bupropion, it may be possible for your GP to switch you to a different medication so that it is safe for you to have both. At least fourteen days should elapse between discontinuation of one drug and the start of the other. If you have a seizure while taking bupropion, you must stop the medication and inform your GP.

Other possible side effects include allergic reactions, which can in rare cases be severe. If you have a severe allergic reaction soon after starting bupropion you must stop taking it, even though it is often difficult to pin down exactly what it is you are sensitive to. Some people may suffer a milder allergic reaction. In this case, discuss your concerns with your doctor. It may be wise to stop the drug and see if the symptoms disappear.

More common side effects include insomnia, dry mouth, agitation, depression or stomach upsets. These are not serious and usually settle down within a week or two. If you experience some side effects but also notice clear benefits you need to decide how much discomfort you are willing to put up with in order to quit smoking. It is worth bearing in mind that many of the side effects are also symptoms of nicotine withdrawal so your discomfort might not even be due to the bupropion.

There has been intense media interest in bupropion and much of the coverage has been irresponsibly alarmist, such as linking the sudden deaths of some young people with bupropion. However, in reality no link between bupropion and sudden death has been established when Zyban is used in accordance with safety guidelines. The sad truth is that sometimes people – even young, apparently healthy people – die suddenly and unexpectedly. This risk is higher among smokers. Naturally when a family is devastated by the sudden death of a loved one the immediate response is to try to find answers and to understand why this terrible thing has happened. If the person had recently started taking a new drug, then the drug is likely to be blamed. This is entirely human, but also illogical. In the attempt to discover whether a drug increases the risk of sudden death, single occurrences do not tell us very much. We need to look at bigger numbers. There have been exhaustive efforts to verify the safety of bupropion. Studies have looked at hundreds of thousands of people to see whether instances of death occur more frequently among those taking bupropion than among other people. The answer is no. Rates of sudden death among bupropion users are no higher than rates of sudden death in the general population. No link has been found between these tragic events and bupropion.

The other factor to bear in mind when deciding whether bupropion is for you or not is that smoking itself is highly dangerous. When you consider that smoking causes 120,000 deaths per year in the UK, there is absolutely no comparison between the tiny risks of bupropion and the huge risks of continuing to smoke.

using bupropion

The course of bupropion is eight weeks long. One tablet a day should be taken for the first six days, then two tablets a day for the rest of the course. If you experience uncomfortable side effects then continue with one tablet a day. The drug takes a few days to reach maximum levels in your bloodstream, so you should wait until the second week of taking the drug before you stop smoking. Some people find that their cigarettes are less and less satisfying as the days go by, and that by quit date they are quite happy to give up. Other people do not notice any difference in their experience of smoking, but have fewer withdrawal symptoms and cravings when they stop. At the end of the eight-week course, you should have been a non-smoker for about six weeks. By this time most nicotine withdrawal is complete, and coming off the bupropion should not be a problem. If you suddenly experience intense cravings again, then these are probably due to psychological factors, and we shall deal with them in the next chapter.

People who use bupropion for several weeks often find that towards the end of the course they forget to take their tablets for several days and do not even notice the difference. This makes sense because by this stage of quitting you will have very little, if any, nicotine left in your system.

However, some people view the tablets as having mythical and magical properties and expect to be swamped with cravings as soon as the course ends. And, surprise surprise, this is exactly what happens. The problem is not the bupropion, or the nicotine. It is the mind. NRT and bupropion can really help you get off nicotine. But staying free involves more than simply getting rid of the physical dependence. You need to get rid of the psychological dependence too. The importance of this was neatly captured by a member of one of my groups. 'That Zyban is bloomin' awful,' he said. 'It makes my cigarettes taste terrible. I had to stop taking it so I could enjoy a fag again!'

the nicotine vaccine – the answer???

The promise of a simple injection to 'cure' nicotine addiction is hugely appealing. Some treatments may be available within five years. Can it really be that easy? Well no, not really…

The aim of the vaccine is to prevent nicotine from reaching the brain. If nicotine does not get to the brain, then it won't affect the person – it will be like smoking a nicotine-free cigarette, which is not satisfying, and so the person will give up more easily. This is actually a very neat illustration of the fact that a person is smoking for nicotine and nicotine alone. Take that away, then a cigarette that tastes identical and still has all the aspects like handling, flicking ash etc becomes pointless. However there are already ways of preventing nicotine reaching the brain – not smoking, for instance! Or smoking nicotine-free cigarettes.

The trouble is that unless people address psychological dependence they will be in the frustrating position of smoking but not gaining any 'pleasure and satisfaction' from their cigarettes – just like my Arctic cigarettes, in fact. So they either remain resentfully abstinent, or they will stop the treatment.

chapter summary

- Angle 1 is nicotine addiction.

- NRT doubles your chance of success.

- NRT is in itself addictive, so take care to use it purely to help you overcome physical dependence, and beware the risk of developing psychological dependence if you use it for too long.

- Patches are the least likely to cause this problem.

- Bupropion (Zyban) may be even more effective than NRT.

- Bupropion is not addictive, but is associated with some health risks.

- Bupropion is available only on prescription.

- Certain types of medical history (e.g. any seizures) increase the risks of bupropion and doctors will not prescribe it in these cases.

- For most people the health risks of bupropion are tiny compared to the risks of continued smoking.

Overcoming Angles 2 & 3: Psychological Dependence & Habit

By now you should be feeling that life as a non-smoker is something positive rather than something negative. Many people enter a quit attempt feeling utterly miserable at the thought of everything they are giving up. The beliefs that have developed over years make them think of cigarettes as something helpful, pleasurable or necessary. These beliefs are untrue. Giving up smoking is nothing more than giving up the need to smoke.

The need to smoke is a time-consuming and expensive nuisance at best, and at worst leaves you climbing the walls with desperation. It ranges from the slightly on-edge feeling you get when you are at a dinner party and no one else has lit up, to the restless anxiety of someone who has run out of fags on the motorway and is late for a meeting but needs to stop anyway to buy some more, to the frantic need that drives you out at 3 a.m. in a blizzard to get fags, to the utter desperation that leads you to smoke through a hole in your neck on the fire escape of the hospital ward, 15 hours after surgery.

The only reason you smoke is that you need to. And all that the cigarette achieves is to stop you needing to – for an hour or so. This need never dies. It continues getting stronger and stronger and stronger until you die – or quit. You will never stop smoking without making a deliberate and conscious effort to do so. Do not waste your time hoping that one day you will just not want to any more. The fact is, you already do not want to, but you are an addict so you have to, no matter how inconvenient or horrible. And that will never change until you stop being an addict.

I finally gave up smoking ten years ago, after many many failed attempts. Even though I had quit on many previous occasions, this time really was different. In all my earlier quit attempts I assumed that smoking was a pleasure and made me feel good, but that it was unhealthy and so I needed to quit. Smoking scared me, but I also felt as if I could not manage without it. Every few months I would make another quit attempt, and sometimes these would last a few weeks. When I got through the first few weeks I tended to find that I was coping okay without smoking – most of the time – but there would still always be situations when I suddenly felt as if I was missing out, and I had cravings again. Inevitably I would tell myself that the odd smoke now and again did no harm, and I would get hooked again. It would then take me months to psych myself up for another attempt.

When I eventually quit properly, I saw smoking for what it really was. At home alone, I took a cigarette out of the packet and was just about to light up when I had that moment of clarity I described earlier (see page 96). It was so powerful and compelling that suddenly I could

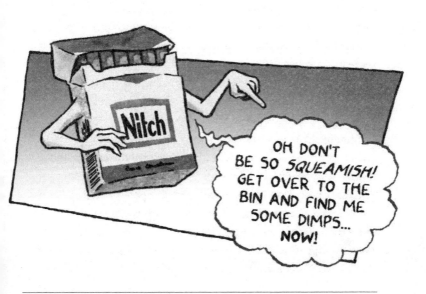

OH DON'T BE SO *SQUEAMISH!* GET OVER TO THE BIN AND FIND ME SOME DIMPS... **NOW!**

see what a miserable existence smokers have. There was nothing good about smoking, it just stopped you feeling bad. But the only reason you feel bad is because you smoke. The only solution – quit and be free.

Key Concept

Smokers don't understand the drive to smoke, so they develop positive beliefs about smoking that provide an explanation.

Some people experience a similar eye-opening flash and quit abruptly with no problem. In my groups these people leave the session saying, 'That's it, never again,' and stop smoking there and then. However, for most people it is not as simple or quick as that, so do not panic if you still feel worried about quitting. Most people gradually come to realise how smoking really works, and the longer they abstain, the more clearly they can see this reality. Nothing clouds your thinking like addiction, so until you are physically free, you are likely to find it hard to grasp fully how great you will feel to be shot of smoking. But you *will* feel great, and you *will* feel free.

Use the worksheets at the end of the chapter to help you overcome Nitch's propaganda.

When you first stop there will be certain situations that are particularly difficult. This is because you will have been conditioned to see smoking as pleasurable or helpful in those situations. Conditioning is a well-understood process. To overcome habitual smoking you need to break all your associations between smoking and other parts of your life, and allow the conditioning to fade away. The tips discussed in Chapter 7 can speed up this process. You may also find it helpful to learn some coping strategies to deal with the temporary difficulties involved in killing Nitch. These include distraction, relaxation techniques and meditation.

distraction

If you have a craving and need something to take your mind off it, try any or all of the following:

- Count backwards from 100 in 7s (100, 93, 86 and so on).
- Think of capital cities beginning with A,B,C right through to Z.
- Wear a rubber band around your wrist and flick it. (Sounds weird but it does sometimes help!)
- Play a favourite song.
- Go and do something else.

relaxation techniques

When smoking cessation advisers suggest that you learn relaxation techniques, the implication is that smoking is relaxing, so when you stop you need an alternative. As we have seen, this is totally untrue. However, learning to relax can help deal with the period of nicotine withdrawal. And learning effective ways to relax can benefit everyone, smoker or non-smoker.

If you are breathing properly you will be using your diaphragm and not your ribs (intercostal muscles). Check this by lying on the floor or sitting upright in a chair with your feet flat on the floor and your back straight. Place your hands fingertip to fingertip over your belly button and breathe in slowly. Your fingers should come apart slightly.

Learning a quick relaxation exercise to reduce tension in your body and to let go of anxiety can be very helpful when you are quitting. Practise the exercises when you are relaxed before trying to use them when you are tense or anxious.

First say 'I am in control' or any other phrase that is positive and calming. Mentally run through your body from head to toe bringing your awareness to each part of the body in turn and letting any tension go. Relax your head, face, eyes, mouth, tongue, jaw, neck, shoulders, chest, and continue right down to your toes. Breathe out, imagining that you are breathing out tension and anxiety. Breathe in slowly, allowing your belly to soften and rise, and imagine breathing in pure white light. With a few repetitions you will feel the tension draining away from your body. Repeat this a few times until you feel calm and relaxed. With practice you will be able to do this quick calming technique when you are walking around or even talking.

meditation

A few years ago I was working in an adult mental health department. The department waiting list included many people who had serious problems with anxiety. While they were waiting for individual treatment, I taught them all either a relaxation exercise, or a type of meditation called Mindfulness of Breathing. I then compared their effectiveness.

I was testing out the idea that meditation would be better at relieving anxiety than straightforward relaxation, because meditation includes your mind, not just your body. In meditation you physically relax your body while at the same time learning to quieten your mind. This is very helpful in anxiety since anxiety generally involves fretting and worrying about things in the future. Learning to stay focused on the here and now is an extremely useful skill.

Another helpful aspect of meditation is that it helps people learn to accept negative emotions calmly and then gently to let those emotions go. In meditation you are aware of exactly how you are feeling, and you simply let yourself feel those emotions, without trying to push them away. Then slowly you focus on your breathing and the negativity drifts away. My research showed that both relaxation and meditation work well to help people cope better with anxiety, but that meditation was more effective.

More recently there has been a lot of additional research into meditation which has shown that it reduces the risk of developing depression and anxiety in people who have had these sorts of problems in the past. This meditation is a fundamental part of Buddhist practice but when used in the context of the NHS, it is separate from any spiritual or religious dimension. You do not need to have any religious beliefs or interests in order to benefit from mindfulness meditation.

In Mindfulness of Breathing meditation first find a comfortable place to sit or kneel. You can sit in a chair keeping your back straight. Or you can kneel astride a big pile of cushions. Try to sit straight and balanced. This takes some practice, so feel free to experiment. Set a timer to go off every four or five minutes. Or record a bell chiming every four or five minutes on a blank tape and play it. Or buy one of the many Mindfulness of Breathing tapes readily available. For a few moments, concentrate on relaxing all parts of your body. Run through your body from head to toe bringing your awareness to each part in turn and letting any tension go. Be aware of any feelings and thoughts you may have. Slowly bring your attention onto your own breathing. Do not alter the rhythm of the breathing. Just notice the differences in each breath. You are now ready to start stage 1.

In stage 1 concentrate on each breath as it enters the body and leaves, enters and leaves. To help deepen your focus on the breath, mentally count one number after every out breath up to ten, then start again from one. That is, breathe in, breathe out and count 1; breathe in, breathe out and count 2, breathe in, breathe out and count 3 and so on.

What you will find almost immediately is that your attention will wander. When you notice that this has happened, gently return your focus to the breathing. Do not worry about how far or for how long your attention has wandered. Do not worry if you have forgotten to start counting from one again when you reached ten and have counted up to fifty! Just gently return your attention to the breathing. Your mind will wander many times during the practice. Do not get irritated, and do not worry that you are 'doing it wrong'.

After four or five minutes, when your timer or bell chimes, you move onto stage 2: in this stage you count just prior to each in breath – count 1, breathe in, breathe out; count 2 , breathe in and breathe out and so on.

When the bell chimes again you progress to stage 3. In this stage you stop counting but simply focus on the breath as it moves in and out of your body.

When the bell chimes again you enter the fourth and final stage. In this stage, narrow your focus down to the touch of the breath as it enters and leaves the body. Be aware of the slight sensations around your nose and upper lip as the air moves across it. When the bell chimes again, slowly bring your meditation practice to an end: relax your concentration. Open your eyes but keep them lowered initially, then gradually look around and re-orientate yourself. At the same time come out of your meditation posture, perhaps with a few gentle stretches.

chapter summary

• Overcoming Nitch's propaganda can take time and patience.

• Overcoming habits can also take time, so don't panic if things feel a little difficult at first.

• Learning relaxation and meditation techniques can be very helpful.

Worksheet 1

Imagine you have *stopped* smoking. Listed below is a number of different situations. Imagine that you are struggling with your quit attempt and so in these situations you have the thoughts described. In each box write down how these sorts of thoughts would make you feel. The first two have been done for you.

Situation	Thoughts	Feelings
Sitting in a pub. Seeing a smoker light up with a satisfied sigh.	Lucky git, he gets to smoke. I bet he's really relaxed. I can't relax without a smoke. It's not fair.	Miserable, jealous, deprived, frustrated
Waking in the morning on quit date.	How will I survive today? It's going to be terrible.	Anxious, dreading it.
The first evening of a holiday.	I can't believe I'm not allowed to smoke. It will ruin the holiday.	
At work struggling with something.	I can't concentrate. I need a fag. I'll never get this done otherwise.	
At home in the evening with the 'I want a cigarette' feeling.	I'm dying for a cigarette. I can't cope with this.	

○ ○

Now repeat the exercise with the following thoughts

Situation	Thoughts	Feelings
Sitting in a pub. Seeing a smoker light up with a satisfied sigh.	He has no choice but to smoke. He will also be smoking tomorrow morning, the next day and the day after that. Look at him squinting away from the smoke. It looks really uncomfortable. I don't have to do that any more.	Relief to be free of it. Pleased with myself for not smoking.
Waking in the morning on quit date.	Don't panic. I never smoked till lunchtime anyway. Withdrawal symptoms aren't that bad – remember the week I spent in hospital?	Calmer, more motivated.
The first evening of a holiday.	Focus on the good things here. Sunshine, cold beer/wine, friends. I'm going to have a great time.	

Situation	Thoughts	Feelings
At work struggling with something.	Nitch is distracting me. If I feed him today he will distract me tomorrow and for ever. This distraction will pass soon.	
At home in the evening with the 'I want a cigarette' feeling.	Nitch is winding me up. He is starving and is complaining. Cigarettes cause these horrible feelings. If I ignore it or just accept it soon Nitch will be dead and I will be free.	

The aim of this worksheet is to teach you the importance of your thoughts. Thoughts strongly affect feelings. So to feel positive and confident, you need to think positively and confidently.

The next step is for you to identify your own negative thoughts. You need to recognise the little 'Nitchisms' that creep into your mind, making you feel anxious or miserable. Then you need to know how to replace the Nitchisms with more positive and realistic thoughts. The next two worksheets help you do this.

○ ○ ○ ○ ○ ○ ○ ○ ○ ○ ○ ○ ○ ○ ○ ○ ○ ○ ○ ○

Worksheet 2

Use these worksheets to identify your own Nitch-speak, and to
challenge it. On the first sheet write down the sorts of things Nitch
might say. On the second sheet, write down more positive thoughts
that will help you think and feel differently about not smoking. Think
of situations you expect to find difficult. Arm yourself with some
positive statements that you can use when you are in those situations.
(Photocopy the pages so you have several examples and fill them in
whenever you feel you are struggling.)

Situation	Thoughts	Feelings

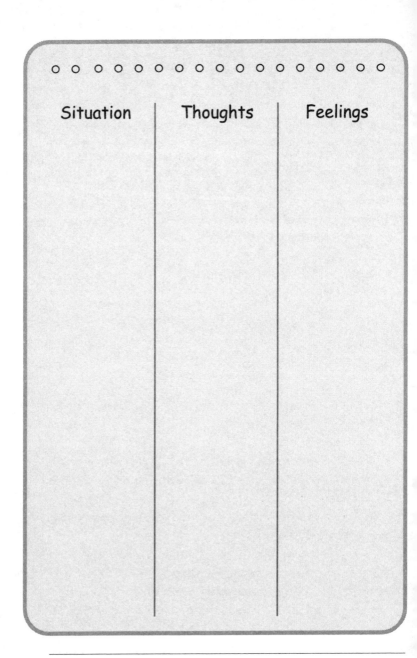

Situation	Thoughts	Feelings

Benefits of Quitting

By now I hope you will feel that there are no good reasons to carry on smoking. So now we can turn to the other side of the coin – all the excellent reasons for quitting. The following facts about smoking are frightening. Smokers do not like to think about the facts of smoking because, naturally, they become anxious and scared by the appalling costs. If you are about to quit, then knowing these facts can help spur you on. If you feel that the facts will just panic you then skip the next section and read 'Health benefits of quitting' instead. Later on in your quit attempt, come back to this section to discover all the dreadful things that are now much less likely to happen to you!

health risks of smoking

- Smoking is the single biggest preventable cause of death and illness in the UK.
- Half of all lifelong smokers will die from their smoking.
- Those who die of smoking-related disease lose on average sixteen years of life.
- Smoking is responsible for 84% of deaths from lung cancer.
- Smoking is responsible for 83% of deaths from lung diseases such as bronchitis and emphysema.
- Smokers have more than twice as much chance of having a heart attack as non-smokers.
- Smoking kills over 120,000 people in the UK every year. That is thirteen people every hour of every day.
- Smoking causes cancers of the lung, mouth, larynx, breast, oesophagus, bladder, kidney, stomach, cervix and pancreas.

- Tobacco harms almost every living tissue in the body that it comes in contact with.
- 7,000 deaths by stroke each year are caused by smoking.
- Smoking is linked to asthma and brittle bone disease.
- Smoking in pregnancy increases your risk of miscarriage by 27%. It also increases your risk of infant illness and low birth weight.
- Smoking is the main contributor to cot death.
- Smoking increases risks of impotence and infertility.
- Smoking doubles your risk of going blind.

It is wonderful that you can avoid these horrendous risks by quitting, but the news is even better than that. You do not have to wait decades to benefit from stopping smoking. You can benefit immediately.

health benefits of quitting

Within 20 minutes
Your blood pressure and pulse return to normal.

Within 8 hours
Carbon monoxide (CO) levels in your bloodstream halve. CO robs your body of oxygen. Smokers therefore have problems with breathing and with circulation. Oxygen makes your blood bright red. CO turns it into a dull greyish colour which is why smokers have grey complexions. As soon as CO levels drop you will look and feel much better.

Within 24 hours
CO levels return to normal. Your lungs start to clean themselves. You may develop a cough. This is just a sign that

your body is undergoing a spring clean, and will be far healthier when this process is complete. Smoking sometimes damps down coughing – but coughing is essential to keep your airways clear. Artificially suppressing this reflex is dangerous to your health.

Within 48 hours
Nicotine has all gone.

Within 72 hours
Your breathing becomes easier and your airways clearer. You have more energy.

Within 2–12 weeks
Your circulation improves and you feel fitter.

Within 3-9 months
Your lung function increases by up to 10%. You have fewer coughs and less wheezing.

Within 1 year
You have halved your risk of heart disease.

Within 2 years
Your risk of a heart attack is now the same as for a lifelong non-smoker.

Within 5-15 years
Your risk of stroke is now the same as for lifelong non-smoker.

Within 10 years
You have achieved a 50% reduction in the risk of lung cancer.

How to Quit

NOTE: If you have glanced through the front of the book and eagerly turned straight to this chapter, well, I am glad you are so keen, but please don't go any further till you have read the preceding chapters. You will not be able to follow these steps without reading and understanding the earlier part. Be patient!

1 Make sense of the book

If you can follow the logic of what you are reading and see how it applies to your smoking you are well on the way, even if you are still nervous of quitting. Re-read any relevant sections to make sure you understand before reading any further.

2 Challenge your thinking

Before you quit, listen out for 'Nitchisms' and challenge them. By 'Nitchisms' I mean the doubts and questions Nitch puts into your head. Review Chapter 5 on propaganda and try to catch yourself making thinking errors. Do not just accept what you think. Thoughts stem from beliefs and attitudes and may not be true. Question what you think and if you notice errors correct them. Draw up worksheets like the ones at the end of Chapters 5 and 10 to help you:

- Identify your thoughts
- Identify the links between the thoughts and your uncomfortable feelings
- Develop alternative thoughts

3 Choose whether or not you want to use NRT or bupropion

If so, choose which product.

4 Plan a quit date

Your quit date is one of the most important days of your life. You will be making a huge decision that will profoundly affect your future health and happiness. Do not just drift into a quit date. Take some time to think seriously about your two alternative futures: the smoking one and the non-smoking one.

Life as a smoker means living with Nitch. It means having to smoke whether you want to or not, no matter how inconvenient. It means experiencing the stress of nicotine withdrawal day in and day out. It means being controlled by the need to smoke. It means having to think about smoking, plan for smoking and find ways of smoking any time and everywhere. It means having to pay for cigarettes whether or not you can really afford them. It means living in fear of the consequences. And it probably means gradually worsening health, leading to devastating diseases and premature death.

Life as a non-smoker means freedom from all that. Life as a non-smoker means no longer playing host to Nitch. It means that smoking will simply not matter. You will not need to think about it, plan life around it, pay for it and die for it.

Think about the two futures, and make a clear choice. Once you have made it, *never doubt it*.

5 Set a quit date

Once you have made the clear and committed decision to quit, then you move from planning a quit date to actually setting one. If you are using NRT, then you will quit on the day you start using the product. Choose a day of the week that you feel will give you the best chance of success. Think about your smoking. Do you smoke more at work or at the weekend? When are the biggest danger periods likely to be? When you have chosen your date, make sure you stick to it. If you start allowing doubts to get the better of you at this early stage, you will struggle later on.

If you are using bupropion, then choose a day in the second week of the treatment.

When you have your quit date, pay close attention to your thoughts and feelings. Use the worksheets in Chapter 10 to help you address any anxieties you may have.

6 Stock up on the items you want to help you quit
These might include relaxation tapes, a meditation tape, sugar free gum, lots of water to flush out your system, fruit and fruit juice to stave off constipation (a common symptom after quitting), a notepad and pen for you to do the thoughts–feelings exercise described in point 2 above if you find yourself struggling.

7 Practice your relaxation techniques or the Mindfulness of Breathing (see Chapter 10)
The more skilled you become in both these practices, the more benefit you gain from them.

8 Smoke normally until you reach your quit date
When you want a cigarette, be conscious of what that feels like. Many people do not find the feeling of wanting a cigarette unpleasant – because they know they are about to have one. So when you want a cigarette, imagine not being able to have one. The feeling then becomes uncomfortable. Say to yourself, 'This feeling of wanting a cigarette is Nitch. Nitch makes me feel bad. Smoking is about living with these uncomfortable feelings, quitting is about being free of them.'

Become increasingly aware of the drive to smoke. Remind yourself that this feeling is anxiety which triggers off a faulty danger signal. Picture smoking as resetting a faulty signal – which will go off at full volume next time it is triggered. Now picture ignoring the signal and letting it fade away and sputter out, like a flat battery. Practise this visualisation regularly.

9 Get rid of smoking-related materials

The night before quit date, after your last cigarette, throw away all smoking-related materials such as ashtrays and lighters as well as any remaining cigarettes. If you find this incredibly anxiety-provoking it is important to question why. What thoughts and assumptions are giving rise to this anxiety? See the worksheets at the end of the chapter to help you.

If you still feel anxious, and think that throwing cigarettes away will make it harder for you to quit, then put them somewhere out of sight. At the end of the first week of quitting, when you have proved you don't need them, throw them away.

Some people like to keep cigarettes around in order to feel power and control over the cigarettes. This is fine. The problem is not so much keeping them, as the reasons for keeping them. If you feel strong and defiant, then keep them. But if you feel anxious and want them around 'just in case', then it is important to get rid of them.

10 Stick to your quit date

Even if doubts persist, *stick to your quit date*. Many people find that their imagination is worse than the reality. Remember that if you are panicking, it is your *thoughts* that are making you panic – not the reality. Do not 'catastrophise' quitting.

11 Quit with confidence

Banish doubt. Never question this decision. Think about how young children respond to different ways of saying 'no'. If parents say 'no' in a way that is clear and consistent, then toddlers accept it with little more than a murmur. If the parents mumble, 'No, almost certainly not, not now anyway, well, we'll see,' then you will get no end of earache until you have given in. Nitch is the same. No must always mean no. Whenever the thought pops into your mind, shout '*No*' at yourself, then let it go. Use distraction. Force your mind onto something else. Do not argue with yourself. Just say, '*No.*'

12 Save cigarette money

Make a 'cash not ash' money box and put it somewhere clearly visible. Each day put in what you would have spent on cigarettes. It is amazing how quickly the money builds up. Plan what you will do with your first £20, £50 and £100. Work out how quickly you'll reach these milestones with the worksheet at the end of this chapter.

13 Break down the conditioned response

If you have particular rituals or routines, change them. This only needs to be temporary but will help you get rid of the conditioned response quickly. Re-read Chapter 10 for more tips on this.

14 Challenge your thinking after quitting

Continue questioning your thinking and watching out for those thinking errors, like 'Just one won't hurt'. Beware 'accidentally on purpose' giving yourself reasons to smoke. Some people will engineer situations to give themselves an excuse to smoke. Be aware of this risk. If you find yourself scheming in this way, stop.

15 Avoid danger at first

Avoid danger situations if necessary at first, but remind yourself that this is *temporary*. It is important to realise that you are only giving up smoking. You are not giving up everything else you enjoy. In time you will enjoy everything else as much as ever before. Start doing relaxing and sociable things as soon as possible so that you prove to yourself that the links between these situations and smoking fade. As your confidence increases put yourself in more and more 'smoking' situations. It is a good idea to avoid alcohol at first because drinking clouds your thinking and reduces your willpower.

16 Expect and accept cravings

When you experience cravings, think of them as Nitch. A craving is not a command, it is just a feeling. Let it be there. It will go away after a few minutes. At first the desire to smoke will come frequently. Then gradually the cravings become less intense and the time between them gets longer. Picture the danger signal slowly running out of power until it fades away completely. Just like a dodgy television remote, you sometimes get a sputtering of life from something you thought was flat, but as long as you don't recharge it (by smoking) it will die in the end.

As your quit attempt continues, you will be moving closer and closer towards total freedom. However, you may have a bad day after several good days. This does not mean that you are back to square one. Accept that progress will not be totally smooth, and hope for a better day the next day. Mindfulness of Breathing helps you learn to accept negative emotional states calmly. As soon as you do this they then fade away gently. Ironically, trying to block out negative emotion makes it last longer. Mindfulness of Breathing also helps get away from the 'what if' worries that people can have when they are stopping smoking, and helps them focus on the here and now.

17 Keep reading

Re-read relevant sections of this book. Use the chapter summaries to remind you of key points.

18 Use support

Phone the NHS Smoking Helpline: 0800 169 0 169 or check out some of the websites listed on page 217.

19 Keep busy

20 Congratulate yourself – you deserve it!

○ ○ ○ ○ ○ ○ ○ ○ ○ ○ ○ ○ ○ ○ ○ ○ ○ ○ ○

Worksheet 1

Get a piece of paper and a pen. Say out loud (and mean it!):

When I quit I will never smoke again.

Try to work out how you feel about that. Write down the feelings that come over you as you look at and say that statement.

Relief?
Excitement?
Terror?
Depression?
Other?

Feelings...

....

....

....

....

Once you know how you feel, try to understand why you feel that way. Write down the feeling and then write down all the thoughts you have that are making you feel that way.

e.g. **Feeling** Anxiety.
Thoughts How will I cope? Cigarettes have always been there for me.

Can you think of any counter-arguments to the above thoughts? Are you making any thinking errors? Which ones?
If your thoughts about never smoking again are positive, well done.

You are on your way. Try to focus more on the positive thoughts than on the negative ones.

Use the following positive self-statements to get yourself into a more positive frame of mind:

• Quitting will give me confidence because I will have proved I can achieve challenges.

• Quitting will make me proud and give me the courage to attempt other challenges too.

• I never needed cigarettes to cope before I started smoking. There is no reason why I need them to cope now.

• Cigarettes make me feel weak. When I quit I will feel stronger and more in control and will cope better with other problems.

• Smoking is a hassle I don't need or want. I am looking forward to being free of the need to smoke.

Add your own:

-
-
-
-
-
-
-
-
-

Worksheet 2

Kick-start your quit attempt with a dose of motivation.

How much do cigarettes cost you?

        per day....................................
        per week................................
        per month.............................
        per yea...................................
        per decade............................

££

What would you most like to do with:

        £5...
        £25...
        £50...
        £100...
        £250...
        £500...

££

How long would it take to save these amounts?

        £5..
        £25..
        £50..
        £100..
        £250..
        £500..

remember

F reedom	**F** ear
R espect	**A** nxiety
E nergy	**G** uilt
E scape	**S** lavery

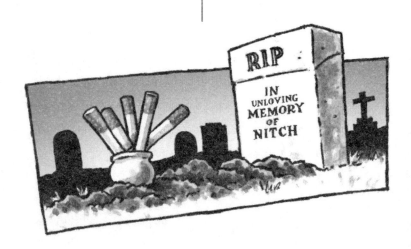

Relapse Prevention: Avoiding the Pitfalls

When you first quit you will be thinking about cigarettes a lot of the time. Thoughts of smoking, cravings and pangs of anxiety will occur frequently. Remember that this is temporary. Remind yourself that the desire to smoke is a chemically induced state of anxiety, plus a load of propaganda, which will stay with you for ever if you smoke and will disappear for ever when you quit.

Key Concept

> **The withdrawal symptoms you struggle with when you are trying to quit will stay with you for ever if you keep smoking and will disappear for ever when you quit.**

Visualise the danger signal slowly winding down till it sputters out for good. Now visualise resetting the danger signal by smoking. Recognise that this just means re-creating the problem. So if you reset the faulty signal you would have to go through the whole process all over again next time you quit. Don't make life harder for yourself. Quitting must mean that you do not smoke *ever*.

Nicotine withdrawal is a chemical process. You have no choice but to go through it, if you want to be free. You must override your danger signals. If you can do this then you will free yourself from Nitch. This difficult time *will* pass. Be patient. You have smoked for a long time. It will take a while for the associations between cigarettes and pleasure or relief to break down. But they will break down – as long as you do not smoke. Cravings can be powerful but they also pass quickly. When one strikes, use distraction. If you can tough it out for three minutes, the chances are it will have gone. Be wary of Nitch and his dirty tricks. He is dying but his propaganda machine may be very much alive. Watch out for Nitchisms and don't be fooled.

Key Concept

Expect and accept cravings. They only last a few minutes.

Over time you will find that you are thinking about cigarettes less and less often. Cravings will become less intense and occur less frequently. Soon you will be going for several hours without thinking about smoking. Later still, you will start going for whole days without thinking about or craving cigarettes. You are still likely, however, to have pangs in certain high-risk situations such as parties, holidays or times of particular stress.

A few weeks down the line, things will be much easier and you may rarely think about smoking at all. You may feel that it was very hard work, or you may feel surprised and delighted by how easy stopping was. You may now be feeling very confident that there is no way that you are ever going to be trapped by smoking again.

This can be a very dangerous time… If you are sensible you will think, 'I am free. I will never smoke again.' But all too often people instead start thinking, 'I've cracked it. I'll never get hooked again. So I can just have the odd one!'

just one cigarette

Nitch's propaganda machine is still waiting for the opportunity to persuade you to smoke again. Giving you a false sense of security is one way of doing that, letting you think that since you have stopped for a while, it is now safe for you to smoke the odd one here or there.

Most people who quit end up back on cigarettes. This is especially true of people who 'dabble'. Even people who did not find it that hard to quit end up trapped again. When you go back to smoking, which cigarette do you blame? The first one you bought? The first one you smoked alone? The first one you smoked in the morning? No! *It was simply the first one!*

Key Concept

Being a non-smoker means not smoking – ever. Every relapse starts with JUST ONE CIGARETTE.

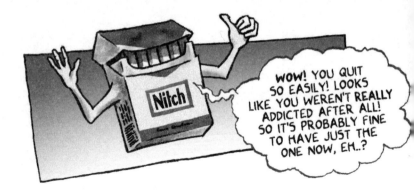

the quantity/ frequency principle

That first cigarette feels safe because smoking is no longer particularly important to you. Imagine you quit smoking eight weeks ago. The first few days of thinking constantly about cigarettes are a distant memory. Over the weeks, you found yourself thinking less and less about them. Whole days can go by without you thinking about smoking. You wake up in the morning and do not need to smoke. You are fine during the day at work. Most evenings are fine too. You feel relaxed and confident. However, there are still occasions where the desire to smoke hits you again. Perhaps these occur when you are at a pub or a party, or when smoking friends visit you.

Having a cigarette on one of those occasions feels quite safe. After all, you barely even think about smoking any more, and just one won't hurt will it?

Yes. *Because the only reason you are in the happy position of hardly ever missing cigarettes, is that **you have not had any.***

As soon as you smoke, everything changes. Instead of being

someone who has not smoked for eight weeks, you are now someone who has smoked recently. You may feel a little concerned about the smoking, and decide to stop again. A few days later you find yourself in a similar situation to the one in which you previously smoked. You tell yourself that you smoked safely last time you were in this situation, so you can have another one. The **frequency** of smoking has gone from zero to one (i.e. you smoke in that one situation only).

Once you are smoking in a particular situation (such as Saturday night) the **quantity** of cigarettes smoked in that situation also rises. Instead of having one, you may have four or five.

You then find yourself thinking about smoking and missing cigarettes in a second situation, similar to the first one. For example, Friday nights. Soon enough you have one on a Friday. The **frequency** of smoking goes up to two situations. Very quickly, smoking on Fridays becomes acceptable in your mind, and the **quantity** of cigarettes smoked on a Friday increases too. Now you may be smoking quite freely over the weekend.

As a result, you now find yourself thinking about smoking, and missing cigarettes on every occasion you go out. So you smoke the odd one during the week, when you are out socially. The **frequency** has gone up again. Once this new 'rule' for when you are allowed to smoke has developed, the **quantity** of cigarettes smoked when out socially also increases. So now you may be smoking three or four nights a week. If you are smoking three or four nights a week, you start thinking about cigarettes and missing them every night. Eventually you smoke one evening when you are relaxing at home. Soon you will be smoking every evening. And if you are smoking every evening, you will start thinking about cigarettes and missing them at lunchtimes. Have you spotted the pattern? The more you smoke, the more you want to smoke. The less you smoke, the less you want to smoke. If you never smoke, the desire to smoke will eventually completely disappear, but if you smoke occasionally, the desire to smoke will increase.

The only way to be a non-smoker is not to smoke. *Ever*!

Key Concept

The quantity/frequency principle says that the situations you smoke in and the amount that you smoke in those situations increases over time.

Do not take it 'one day at a time'. Smoking is not a one-day-at-a-time kind of thing. In fact thinking realistically about the future can be powerfully motivating. Smoking is a lifelong chain that never weakens and never breaks unless you break it. The only way to break the chain is to accept that you cannot control smoking. You do not smoke because you want to, or you choose to, or you like to. You smoke because you *have* to. It is not a free choice. One cigarette leads to the next and the next and the next and the next. The only way to break the chain is to stop smoking completely and permanently.

If you do relapse, it is very important that you do not give yourself false hope by telling yourself that smoking the odd one now and again will do you no harm. Instead you need to be honest with yourself. Remind yourself that smoking is not something that can be controlled. The only way to be free of smoking is not to smoke. Ever. If you have lapsed you need to learn what you can from the lapse, restate your aim of never smoking and stop again immediately.

learning from relapse

Many smokers have small slip-ups in the first few days and weeks of quitting. But just because it's common doesn't mean that it doesn't matter. Remember, 100% of people who go back to smoking start with just one! If you have smoked one or two cigarettes in one or two places, do not kid yourself that this is fine. I'd love to be able to say, 'Well never mind, you've done really well anyway' (even though you have), because unfortunately these small slips really do matter.

If you slip up there is an immediate impact on all three angles of the Smoking Triangle:

- You re-awaken Nitch and reset the faulty danger signal.
- You fail to allow the conditioning to fade so you don't break the association between cigarettes and pleasures or benefits.
- You reawaken cognitive dissonance because you have the thoughts 'I'm quitting' and 'I'm smoking' at the same time. This in turn greatly increases your risk of believing Nitch's propaganda. So you strengthen psychological dependence too.

Don't make life harder for yourself!

The biggest problem you are likely to face is the newly reawakened cognitive dissonance. You will want to believe that it's okay, so you may say things like 'Just one won't hurt' or 'I'll only smoke occasionally, and it won't really matter' or even 'I've done so well so I deserve a cigarette to treat myself.' A little further down the line, as it becomes obvious that the 'odd one here or there' is turning into the odd many here and everywhere, cognitive dissonance will get even stronger and you will start wanting to believe that you don't care that much about quitting anyway. Instead of reducing cognitive dissonance by kidding yourself either that the slip doesn't matter, or that you are not that bothered about quitting anyway, you need an alternative way to reduce dissonance – and here it is:

Tell yourself that you made a mistake, which is fine, everyone makes mistakes at times. Tell yourself that the good thing about making mistakes is that you can learn from them. Tell yourself that the only time you will not learn from a mistake is by pretending it wasn't really a mistake after all. The little mistake was smoking. The huge mistake is pretending it does not matter. Remind yourself that you successfully quit up until the relapse so you have proved that you can do it. And *most importantly*, restate your objective firmly. Your goal is to not smoke – ever.

Key Concept

> If you relapse you need to work out why, correct it and stop again immediately.

stress and relapse

When you were smoking, anxiety increased between each cigarette. Every time you smoked, this anxiety would disappear, making you feel a bit better. If life stressed you out, you had two problems:

1 The real problem in your life
2 The need to smoke

Your overall stress levels were a combination of these two things. Your body could not tell the difference, since Nitch stress mimics ordinary stress. Smoking therefore reduced these overall stress levels, making you feel better. This is why people are more likely to smoke when they are stressed and why they experience cigarettes as helpful.

It is crucial to realise that they only feel helpful if you need the nicotine. Now that you are no longer a nicotine addict, smoking will no longer help reduce your overall stress levels. But it can be very difficult to remember this fact when you are in a crisis.

If you have not smoked for a while, and are nicotine free, any stress you experience will come from life, not from nicotine withdrawal. Therefore any solutions need to come from life too. But when you are in a crisis it is the most natural thing in the world to want to reach out for something to help you feel better. As an ex-smoker, if you experience something terrible, such as a bereavement, unemployment or serious illness, you are likely to remember smoking as something that helped you cope. You are likely, therefore, to be tempted to smoke again. The trouble is that your memory is playing tricks on you. When you are anxious you remember vividly that in the past these feelings were relieved by smoking. But only because your anxiety was caused by smoking.

Think back to previous relapses. If you turned to cigarettes at a time of crisis, what were they like for you? Many people don't even know, because they are in the middle of a crisis and have other things on their mind. But those people who can remember say the first cigarette did nothing at all to help. But having had the first, they had to have the second, and the third…

When I was in the middle of one of my many quit attempts, my husband was involved in a serious accident. I was waiting with friends at the hospital for news of his condition. My friend (who was a lifelong non-smoker) went to the shop and bought me some cigarettes. At a time like that, worrying about my own health seemed ridiculous, so I smoked them. I have no recollection of what the first two or three were like, but smoking is something that hooks you with extraordinary speed, so by the next morning I was hooked on cigarettes again. My husband was fine, and I was a nicotine addict again. For the next week or so, while he recovered in hospital, I had to keep leaving his bedside to go down eighteen floors to stand outside in the snow to smoke. This was not helpful!

When you are stressed by life, cigarettes change nothing about the reality of your situation. You have to deal with whatever it is that life is throwing at you, whether or not you smoke. If you are a non-smoker, the real issues are the only issues, and smoking cannot help with those. Non-smokers do not think of turning to cigarettes to help them cope. There is no evidence that non-smokers cope less well, just because they are unable to use cigarettes as a crutch. In fact the research shows that non-smokers cope much better with problems and are generally less stressed and happier than smokers.

As an ex-smoker, the first cigarette you have in a crisis will also not make you feel any better. But unfortunately, as an ex-smoker you are likely to have memories of smoking that persuade you that smoking really does help. These memories are very powerful. The second cigarette is also unlikely to help you, but very quickly your dependency reawakens and you start to need cigarettes. Within a few hours of your first cigarette you are likely to be puffing away thinking, 'I really really need these. I cannot possibly cope with this without smoking.' The tragedy is that if you had not had the first one, you would have coped just as well without any of them. But as soon as you reawaken the addiction, then you will need to smoke on top of all your other problems. If you are in a stressful situation, try telling yourself: 'Thank goodness I've quit. At least my real problems are my only problems – in the old days I'd have needed to smoke too.'

Key Concept

Smoking can only reduce the anxiety it causes. It will not help with stress after you have quit.

beware false memories

Memories of cigarettes helping you deal with crises are misleading because the memory is only one half of the story. People remember the relief, the 'aahh' factor, without recalling how stressed and miserable the *need* for the cigarette was. It is therefore crucial to fix firmly in your mind that cigarettes do not do anything to help with stress. Try to think of a time when you were desperate for a cigarette. Remember in as much detail as possible what that felt like. Then if you ever find yourself thinking about the 'aahh' factor, make yourself remember the stress of needing to smoke at the same time. You cannot have one without the other.

Key Concept

> You can't have the 'aahh' factor without the 'aarrgg' factor!

A woman in one of my groups demonstrated this really well. When she first came to see me, she said she could not stop smoking because she had three children under the age of four, and the baby was ill a lot of the time. She therefore needed to spend many hours pacing up and down with the baby in her arms while he cried and cried. This was naturally extremely stressful and distressing. The woman felt that smoking helped her with those stresses. She described how she could feel the need to smoke getting stronger as she paced round the living room with her baby. She did not want to smoke over the baby, but leaving him made her feel guilty. So she would wait till the craving was overwhelming, then she would put the baby in his cot and dash outside for the fastest cigarette possible, before running back in to soothe her child again. Others in the group could see that far from helping her, the need to smoke was an extra hassle that greatly increased her stress, but she was not able to see this herself at first. Eight weeks after quitting she came back to her follow-up appointment and reported how much simpler life was now that she no longer needed to smoke. Instead of three kids *plus* Nitch, she now just had the three kids to worry about. She was coping much better with her stresses than ever before.

Try to remember when you are stressed that being a nicotine addict is expensive, time-consuming and above all stressful. If you have problems in your life, the last thing you should do is add to them by waking Nitch up again.

a note on depression

Cigarettes act on brain pathways. There are chemicals in the brain called Dopamine (DA) and Noradrenaline (NA) which are raised by nicotine. DA and NA are lowered in people with clinical depression. Sometimes people who are depressed find that nicotine has a mild anti-depressant effect, because it raises these levels in the brain. If these people give up smoking, they sometimes find themselves becoming depressed. (Please note that cigarettes do not lift your mood if you are not clinically depressed.) A complicating factor, however, is that many people who are miserable when they quit, are not miserable because of the above process, but because their thoughts about smoking are making them unhappy.

If you are really struggling with your quit attempt, and feel miserable and depressed, it is important to try to identify the root causes of your problems. Ask yourself when the low mood started. If you felt bad before you even quit, then this is clearly not a chemical reaction. If, on the other hand, you felt okay about quitting, but are gradually feeling worse and worse, then it may be that you are slightly depressed. If this is the case, the solution is to treat the underlying depression – not to go back to smoking. Anti-depressant medication raises DA and NA levels more effectively (and much, much more safely) than smoking does. Some people also find St John's Wort helpful. This is widely available without prescription.

It is worth noting that Zyban is an anti-depressant, so for smokers who are depressed or at risk of becoming depressed, Zyban can be particularly useful.

Even if you do not like the idea of medication, diagnosing the problem can make you feel better. Ask your GP for advice. And also note that if you are unhappy about medication for depression, but are tempted to smoke instead to lift your mood, this is rather like someone saying, 'I don't like the idea of injections, so I'll just chop off my arm instead.'

weight gain

For some people, worry about gaining weight prevents them trying to quit. For others, weight gain after quitting makes relapse more likely.

Most people gain a small amount of weight over several months when they quit. This is typically from 5 to 10 pounds and is due to several factors. Understanding these factors helps you to minimise any weight gain.

metabolic changes post-quitting

When you quit, your metabolic rate goes down by a very small amount. Unless you make an equivalent adjustment to how many calories you take in or burn up, you will very slowly gain some weight. Just 100 spare calories a day lead to 1 pound of weight gain a month. On the other hand it is easy to make adjustments of 100 calories to your diet or to burn an extra 100 calories through some exercise. So a little forward planning and effort will prevent this weight gain. Walking a mile burns about 100 calories and will take you about 20 minutes. Try to get into the habit of going for a short walk every day (or indeed a long one!). Use some of your saved smoking money to get gym membership. Buy a pedometer and aim to walk 10,000 steps a day. The huge success of these pedometers shows how motivating having clear targets and instant feedback can be.

increased appetite post-quitting

Sometimes people who are trying to control their weight use cigarettes as a substitute for food. They may smoke a cigarette instead of having a snack, or as an excuse to delay their meals. To overcome this problem you need to recognise that no one ever gains weight by eating when they are hungry (as opposed to eating to fill emotional needs such as loneliness, boredom or stress). People gain weight by eating when they are *not* hungry, or eating too much when they are. If your appetite is better after quitting, don't panic. Eat when you are hungry, but stop once your hunger has been satisfied. If people gain weight after quitting because they are no longer able to use cigarettes instead of eating, it is because they eat past the point of satisfaction, or snack when they are not hungry, not simply because they have an appetite. You need to learn to celebrate hunger and appetite as it means 'Hooray, it's time to eat!'

food tastes better

Far from being a problem, this is one if the wonderful benefits of quitting. You can taste food! When you stop smoking your taste buds and sense of smell recover and long-forgotten tastes from pre-smoking days are reawakened. Many smokers have actually forgotten just how fabulous food smells when not masked by the odour of cigarette smoke. Some smokers fear enjoying food in the same way that they fear hunger and appetite.

However, paradoxically, the more you enjoy your food, the more satisfying it is, and the less you need to eat. Fabulous food satisfies far more than mediocre (or smoke-masked) food, both of which tempt you to eat more and more in an attempt to be satisfied. Eating delicious food in response to genuine hunger satisfies your needs completely. You are doing precisely what your body and mind want you to do. It is a perfect match and so it satisfies perfectly.

no trigger to end meals

Many people immediately light up at the end of a meal, and this signals that eating is over. Without this signal people can eat beyond satisfaction by helping themselves to more even if they have had enough, or by extending the meal further with more courses (a piece of cheese, pudding, a biscuit). To solve this problem you can develop a new signal such as a cup of coffee. Or you can avoid it by plating food up in the kitchen rather than having dishes filled with food on the table tempting you to second helpings, or only cooking what you want to eat.

trying to replace cigarettes

This is the biggest danger to quitters, and the reason for any large weight gain, rather than the 5–10 pound small weight gain discussed above: eating to fill the 'gap' left by smoking. This is a *much* bigger problem for people who quit without addressing psychological dependence. If you quit believing you are giving up a genuine pleasure, then you will feel that you are missing out. You will therefore automatically start looking for other treats to replace the 'pleasure' of smoking, or to give yourself rewards to make up for the loss of cigarettes: 'I'm not allowed to smoke any more, so I'll treat myself to a chocolate bar instead.'

There are several misconceptions embedded in that statement:

• 'I'm not allowed' implies that you are depriving yourself of something you want. You would love to smoke, but you are not allowed to because it is unhealthy and expensive. The truth of the matter is that of course you are allowed to smoke. You are an adult, you can do what you want. Quitting must be an active choice, not a chore undertaken with petulant resignation. Think *liberation* not *deprivation*.

• 'I'll treat myself to ... instead.' This implies cigarettes were a treat. They weren't. They were a necessity and a monumental pain in the rear. You do not need to replace them. Celebrate their disappearance!

• Chocolate is indeed a lovely treat – if you are hungry. But if you are not hungry you need to stop seeing food as a treat. If you want some chocolate, but you are not hungry, then what do you really want? Comfort? Relief from boredom? Something to relax you? Excitement? A reward after a difficult week? Distraction from a craving? Work out what you really want and then meet that need. If you apply the wrong solution (eating chocolate when you are not hungry, for instance) it won't work and then you will simply repeat it in a futile attempt to meet the need.

If you have read this book, you will be far less likely to search for a replacement for smoking. On the contrary, you will be delighted to be free, so it is unlikely that you will gain significant amounts of weight. However, you may still experience some small weight gain due to the other factors mentioned above. Bear in mind that quitting smoking will give you a huge confidence boost. You will feel better, look better, have more energy and feel extremely proud of what you have achieved. Dealing with weight issues is much easier in that frame of mind.

oops, I'm smoking again...

If you have a major relapse and recognise that you are smoking again, take heart! You can learn a lot from relapses and this will help you when you quit again.

- Accept that you are smoking.
- Review how you were doing until you relapsed.
- Remind yourself of any positives that you discovered: for example, that withdrawal was not as bad as you had expected, or that you had stopped thinking about cigarettes a lot of the time.
- *Write these down* – once they have started again, many people forget that they were fine when they stopped.
- Work out what the triggers were.
- Identify any thinking errors that led to cravings or relapse.
- Create a plan for dealing with those triggers differently next time.
- Set another quit date.

a case example

Amy is twenty-eight years old. She stopped smoking by using patches for eight weeks. She did not deal with psychological dependence when she quit, so she thought of smoking as a pleasure that she was giving up for health reasons. She had awful withdrawal symptoms for about a week and then started to feel better. She avoided all social occasions for the first three weeks because she was scared she would smoke again. This made her fed up because she felt she would never really enjoy herself in the same way again. After that she began to go out and was pleasantly surprised by how well she coped with not smoking when she was out with her friends.

Eight weeks after Amy quit, her best friend was turning thirty and Amy was dreading the party. She felt anxious about the high risk of smoking but felt deprived at the thought of going to the party and not smoking. She was certain she would have a miserable night and might ruin it for her friend (who was a smoker).

She made the decision to smoke at the party. She told herself it was only for one night, that she had coped okay with not smoking but that it was such a special occasion that she would not risk ruining it.

She lit her first cigarette with excited anticipation. It was horrible. It tasted foul and it did not satisfy her. She was disappointed but tried another one. This one made her feel slightly sick. An hour later, once she had reached the party, she lit up a third cigarette which was more like she remembered them. After that she chain-smoked and was barely aware that she was smoking at all.

The next morning her clothes stank, her mouth tasted terrible and she had no hesitation in saying, 'Yuck, never again.' However, that evening she experienced cravings again. She decided just to finish off the packet. There were six left. The first cigarette felt very satisfying. She smoked another before bed and smoked two a night over the next two nights.

The third evening she was craving a cigarette. She did not smoke, but had a miserable evening. The next night she arranged to go out to the pub with some smoking friends and cadged a few of theirs. This pattern of occasional smoking with the odd miserable night off cigarettes continued for another fortnight until she went out one evening to buy a packet and accepted she was smoking again.

how could she learn from this?

Remember the plan:

Accept you are smoking

Amy needs to acknowledge that she is back smoking again and needs to regroup for another quit attempt. She shouldn't try to stop again until she feels ready to set another quit date and give the attempt the thought and effort it deserves.

Review how you were doing until you relapsed

Amy needs be honest about what being a non-smoker was actually like, rather than focusing on what she expected or imagined it would be like. What she found was that withdrawal symptoms disappear quite quickly, that she was thinking less and less about smoking and that evenings out were fine without smoking. What she also discovered was that she made negative predictions about what not smoking at a party would be like. These predictions made her feel deprived and miserable. Next time she should therefore concentrate on psychological dependence so that she can have a more positive view of life after smoking.

She discovered that the first cigarette was horrible, which confirms that cigarettes are not really pleasurable in themselves – they just take away Nitch stress. She discovered that Nitch gets his claws into you again very quickly. She discovered that smoking was no big deal, in fact she can barely remember doing it most of the night. She discovered that even if you did not enjoy smoking, you will feel anxious and edgy a few hours after smoking, and this anxiety will lead you to crave cigarettes.

Remind yourself of any positives that you discovered

Amy needs to focus on the positive things that she learned.

Write the positives down
- I coped fine without smoking.
- Even pubs were no problem.
- I overcame nicotine withdrawal without much difficulty.
- My imagination was worse than the reality.

Work out what the triggers were

In Amy's case the trigger was a party. Or to be precise the trigger was a set of beliefs about the party, plus an inaccurate assumption that smoking just the odd one would not lead to full blown relapse.

Identify any thinking errors that led to cravings or relapse

Amy needs to recognise that she tends to assume the worst, even though she actually experienced that going out and not smoking was fine. She also kidded herself that smoking occasionally would be okay.

Create a plan for dealing with triggers differently next time

Amy needs to recall that the first two cigarettes were disgusting anyway.

She needs to remind herself that she *cannot* smoke occasionally.

She needs to address psychological dependence so that she is not tricked by Nitch into misery and stress.

She needs to remember that she was fine as a non-smoker, even in high-risk situations.

Set another quit date

And this time deal with all three angles of the Smoking Triangle.

chapter summary

- After quitting expect and accept cravings.

- Cravings are just the faulty danger signal going off.

- Quitting involves overriding these danger signals.

- Quitting also involves breaking habits. Be patient – you have smoked a long time.

- Nitch will be waiting in the wings hoping for a weak moment to snare you with propaganda.

- Not smoking means never smoking. All relapses start with just one cigarette.

- You will have a memory of smoking reducing your anxiety. It is crucial to remember that smoking only reduced Nitch stress, not stress in real life. Once Nitch is dead, smoking cannot possibly help you.

- If you relapse, work out why, fix it and restate your objective immediately.

- This objective is (of course!) *not smoking ever.*

Social Smokers

By now I hope that the idea of being a so-called 'social smoker' is less attractive to you than it might have been before you started reading. However, some people do desperately cling to the false hope of 'social smoking' and so it is important to explain exactly why this just does not and will not work.

The social smoker is this fabled creature who can 'take or leave' cigarettes, who only smokes on special occasions but never *needs* to smoke, who can 'enjoy' a cigarette every so often but is never out of control. A smoker, in other words, who is choosing when, where and whether to smoke, and who can go without cigarettes with no problem. Therefore he or she can enjoy all the pleasures of smoking with none of the drawbacks. Sounds good? Well, let's take a closer look.

You may know people who are genuinely like this. You may also know people who present themselves and their smoking like this but are kidding you (and themselves).

genuine 'social smokers'

Over 90% of teenagers who smoke four cigarettes will take up regular smoking. This makes nicotine one of the most addictive drugs on earth. However, not everyone does get hooked on nicotine as quickly as that. There is considerable individual variation in the ease with which a person can develop a dependency. Take alcohol for example. Most people can drink moderate amounts with no problem. Quite a lot of people can drink quite heavily without becoming alcoholics. Unfortunately some people are not so lucky, and do become alcoholics on smaller amounts of drink. The addictive processes for smoking are similar. The vast majority of smokers get hooked with astonishing and frightening ease. But there are a tiny minority who can smoke a lot more cigarettes and not develop a dependency. Even these people will get hooked if they smoke enough, but they need to smoke quite a lot before this happens.

People who are lucky enough not to get hooked on smoking (yet) have no idea what smoking is all about. You are not one of these people. It is nothing to do with willpower, skill, practice, superior character or finding the secret of how to smoke socially. It is sheer chance. The social smokers themselves will not realise this and are likely to feel smug and superior. They may try to tell you how to do it. You can't. And nor would they be able to if they were born different. Ignore them. They do not know what they are talking about.

> ## Key Concept
>
> **You cannot learn to control cigarettes. If you have ever struggled to control smoking in the past, you will not be able to control it in the future.**

misleading 'social smokers'

Of the social smokers you think you know, only a tiny, tiny minority are likely to be genuinely not hooked. The others think that they are in control but are in fact mistaken. Many social smokers are people who have smoked heavily in the past. Then they quit for some time. Then they started smoking again, but only small amounts *at first*. And that is the crucial point. People sometimes relapse with an almighty crash and are back on twenty, thirty or forty a day within a week or two of relapsing. However, some people ease more gradually back into the Smoking Triangle. But all are going in the same direction – back to regular smoking. Think back over your own quitting history, or the experiences of people you know. Smoking again after quitting starts with the odd one at a party or pub, then the odd few at the weekends, then the odd one on weekday evenings, then the odd few on weekday evenings, then the odd one at lunchtime and so on.

At each stage of this process the person may feel and believe that he (or she) is in control. After all, the smoker still remembers that he used to smoke within minutes of waking and it is nothing like that now, so he is obviously in control…isn't he?

No!

The reality of all addictions is that the more you do, the more you need to do. In a step by step process, the number of different occasions or situations when you smoke increases, then the amount smoked in those situations increases, then the number of situations increases again and so on.

The reason people think they are in control is because they are smoking (and thinking about smoking) far less than they used to. *But it doesn't stay like that.* In all addictions the more you do the more you do. Social smokers are therefore just people who used to be regular smokers and are on their way back to being regular smokers, but mistakenly assume that things are different this time.

Key Concept

> **Some 'social smokers' are relapsing smokers who are on their way back to full-time smoking.**

You never believed you were getting hooked the first time you got hooked, so perhaps it is not surprising that you do not realise you are getting hooked again. If you meet someone who assures you he is in control, wait six months. You will find he has either quit properly or is smoking regularly again.

Social smokers also tend to underestimate how much they are actually smoking.

Key Concept

Never believe what smokers tell you. Social smokers tend to smoke more than they think they do.

self-controlled social smokers

The exceptions to the above rule are the smokers who want to smoke more than a few each week, but do not allow themselves to. These people set themselves a limit and ruthlessly stick to it.

Perfect solution? Well, actually, no. This is a very difficult option. Occasional smokers are still in the triangle:

- They keep Nitch alive (or they repeatedly resurrect him).
- They fail to break the associations between smoking and social situations, work breaks, pleasure and relaxation.
- They keep psychological dependence going.

The result is that they think about smoking all the time. They live their whole life as if they were in the first week of a quit attempt –

constantly thinking about smoking, experiencing withdrawal symptoms almost all day, and never being free of smoking. And there is no end in sight. They are still feeding Nitch, so Nitch will not die. But he is not being fed enough to satisfy him so it is like being permanently hungry. This is much harder than just quitting completely.

Key Concept

Self-controlled smoking is much harder than total abstinence. It is like permanently being in the first week of a quit attempt.

Why aspire to this? In fact why does anyone do it? Well, the answer, as ever, lies in the beliefs and attitudes of the smoker. Smokers like this have extremely positive views of smoking. And the less they smoke, the more satisfying each cigarette feels, so the more powerful the fundamental misconception is.

The different experience you have of cigarettes at different times is due to how hungry Nitch is at different times. Remember, cigarettes do not change. All that changes is your readiness to have one. If you are chain-smoking you do not want or need to smoke, so when you do smoke it is unpleasant. If you are smoking heavily but not chain-smoking, Nitch is less full, but is still not hungry, so a cigarette is fairly meaningless, but not terrible. But what if you have not smoked for hours? Well, then Nitch is starving and the cigarette feels great. It is at those times that you think, 'I can't live without these.' But the reality remains that the only reason the cigarette was so good was because before smoking it Nitch was making you feel so bad.

Ruthlessly self-controlled smokers are experiencing Nitch misery almost all the time. When they finally allow themselves to smoke it is such a relief. This relief is so powerful that it makes them feel completely unable even to think about giving up cigarettes. So they cannot win. They will never be free, but they have to spend almost all day withdrawing from nicotine. This is not something to aspire to. Your best chance of future happiness and freedom is to accept that you will never smoke again. Ever. That is what being a non-smoker means. This is only a problem if you want to be a smoker.

I know I can never smoke again. This is fine because – guess what – I do not ever *want* to smoke again. The secret of success, therefore, is to get yourself into a frame of mind where being a non-smoker is something you actively want.

what social smoking usually means

Often smoking socially is nothing more than an excuse to justify smoking. People who need to smoke, but do not like to admit this need to themselves, can kid themselves that they are 'just being sociable'. You may come across people who tell you in all sincerity that they only ever smoke a few when they are out – they in fact smoke a packet but then delete most of those cigarettes from their memory, and wonder where on earth all their fags have gone.

Other people go out every night of the week – to give themselves an excuse to smoke. The ability of smokers to delude themselves is hard to exaggerate. When I was studying for my degree, I transferred from one university to another and started at the second university in the second year. I lived alone, seventeen miles away from the campus, I did not know anyone, and everyone in my year knew each other already, so it was hard to make new friends. When I arrived at the university I was ten weeks into another quit attempt, and feeling fairly positive about it. One day soon after getting there, I went to the sports centre to see if I could join any clubs and get to know people that way. I saw a group of lads standing outside the centre having a cigarette. I stopped to have a chat about what they were doing and they said they were climbers about to use the climbing wall and invited me to join them. I readily accepted. They offered me a cigarette. I accepted even more readily, telling myself I was just being sociable.

The next night I happened to find myself outside the sports centre at just the right time for the pre-climbing fag, and accepted another one – again 'just to be sociable'. Now this was totally illogical. I had met them before and did not need to smoke to give myself an excuse to talk to them. I was, in any case, about to spend an hour climbing with them. But reality never gets in the way of a decent excuse to smoke! I spent the rest of the week smoking their cigarettes. Then I started buying my own. I still told myself I was just being sociable. After all, I only smoked with these particular people. It just so happened that I saw them every evening.

I started going on climbing trips at weekends and therefore smoked freely all day and all night when I was away. But I still did not consider myself a 'real' smoker and it was at least two months before I admitted to myself that I was actually a smoker again. Do not pretend you are only smoking to be sociable if the reality is that you are mostly being sociable to let yourself smoke!

Key Concept

Dont kid yourself that you are only smoking to be sociable if in reality you are mostly being sociable to let yourself smoke!

chapter summary

- Some people take longer to get hooked than others.

- Most 'social smokers' are really either relapsing smokers or self-controlled smokers.

- Most people cannot control cigarettes at all.

- Even those who can are never truly free of smoking.

- This is a miserable and difficult option.

- The only way to be truly free is never to smoke – ever.

Beware other smokers

Sometimes smokers find it hard when other people stop smoking. Recognise any of these?

- 'Go on, just have one!'
- 'Here, have one of mine – one won't hurt.'
- 'You haven't smoked in a week, you deserve a treat.'

You may also find people offering you a 'friendly' invite to go outside for a smoke. Sometimes people will even light two cigarettes and hand one to you. If you smoke you belong to a club that is very welcoming and being invited to share is hard to resist. On ITV's *X Factor* in 2005 the presenter Kate Thornton was asked, 'William or Harry?' 'William,' she replied, before pausing. 'No, Harry – he smokes fags,' she decided.

So why are smokers so friendly to each other? And why are they particularly generous with their cigarettes to people who are trying to quit?

The truth is that smokers feel insecure when other people quit. Remember the ostrich syndrome? Smokers are terrified of the implications of smoking and try very hard to ignore, deny or distort these. One effective way of distorting reality is to believe in safety in numbers! If you surround yourself with other smokers it is easier to convince yourself that smoking cannot really be that bad, can it? This is just more of Nitch's propaganda. He will direct your attention to happy, smiling smokers enjoying beers in the pub and then say, 'If smoking really is so bad, why aren't these people more stressed about it? They don't seem to mind, so it must be all right really….'

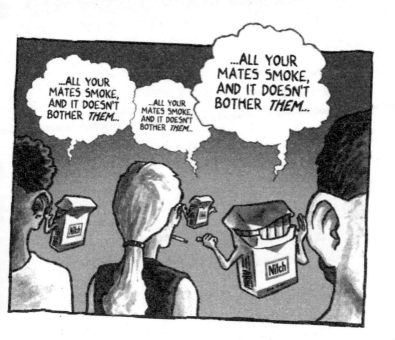

The sense of solidarity among smokers hides insecurity. Smokers may not want you to stop, because this will highlight their own fears. They will try to make you feel jealous and will go on about how much they enjoy smoking or how relaxed they are about their own smoking. This is unlikely to be deliberate, but it can be devastating unless you are aware of it.

Never be envious of smokers. Remember the research – over 90% of people want to stop smoking. No one takes up smoking with the intention of smoking for life. All smokers wish they had never started in the first place.

dealing with smokers

If people try to make you smoke, take a step back to work out why this is happening.

• Does the smoker feel awkward about being the only smoker and want you to help them feel less self-conscious? **If so, this is their problem, not yours**.

• Is your stopping smoking making the smoker feel anxious and insecure? **Their problem, not yours.**

• Does the smoker think that you will become a different person if you quit – and they like you the way you are? **Prove to them that this will not happen. You will still be you, you just won't smoke.**

• Is the smoker genuinely convinced you will be stressed and unrelaxed if you do not smoke? **Reassure them by what you say and how you behave that you are absolutely fine.**

• Does the smoker need you to make them feel better about their own smoking? **Their problem, not yours.**

• Does the smoker worry that you are going to lecture them and become sanctimonious and smug? **Reassure them that you are not bothered by what other people do. You are not turning into an anti-smoking health bore by quitting, you are just quitting.**

miserable ex-smokers

People who quit years ago but still miss cigarettes can be very damaging to your confidence. Nitch will immediately latch onto this and tell you that the misery of quitting is not worth it. But what is really going on for these people?

The simple truth is that if people believed that smoking was wonderful the day they quit, they may well continue to believe the same thing years later. This is a tragedy, because people do not realise that they are missing a false memory. They miss the sense of satisfaction, while failing to remember how miserable the need to smoke made them feel first. They believe that they gave up something that gave them courage, comfort, confidence, concentration and creativity. Something that relaxed them and relieved them. Something that cheered them up when they were miserable, made good times even better, was a friend and constant companion. No wonder they miss it! If cigarettes really did all this, smokers would be more chilled out, relaxed, happy and contented than the rest of us. Research shows the opposite is true.

So why do so many smokers get it wrong?

Because the benefits are costs in disguise!

- Cigarettes stress you out, then take some of that stress away.
- Cigarettes distract you, then give some concentration back.
- Cigarettes get in the way of enjoyment, then let you enjoy yourself again.
- Cigarettes cause misery, then take some of it away.
- Cigarettes rob you of everything – courage, confidence, enjoyment, contentment – then pretend to be enhancing these qualities.

If you meet a miserable ex-smoker just remember that they are missing something that they never had. If you do not believe the propaganda, you will not miss smoking. On the contrary, you will be delighted finally to be free.

chapter summary

• Smokers often find other people quitting quite threatening.

• Smokers prefer 'safety in numbers' and may consciously or unconsciously undermine your quit attempts.

• Some ex-smokers still miss cigarettes. This is because they quit without freeing themselves from Nitch's propaganda.

• This won't happen to you, so don't let it worry you.

• Once you have freed yourself from Nitch both physically and mentally, nothing and no one will ever get in the way of your permanent freedom from smoking.

Congratulations!

16

This is to certify that I,

....

am a non-smoker!

Since quit date on..........................

I have saved £..............................

I will continue to save

£.....................per month

Tick as appropriate

- [ ] I am fitter
- [ ] I am healthier
- [ ] I am less breathless
- [ ] I look and feel younger
- [ ] My skin is rosier
- [ ] My senses of taste and smell have improved
- [ ] I no longer smell like an ashtray
- [ ] I feel more in control
- [ ] My breath is no longer bad
- [ ] My house smells clean and fresh
- [ ] I have more energy
- [ ] My family are proud of me
- [ ] I am very proud of myself!

Other benefits I have noticed

....

....

....

....

References

Chapter 2

1 (page 28)
Russell, M. A. H. (1990) 'The nicotine addiction trap: a 40 year sentence for four cigarettes'. *British Journal of Addiction*, 85, 293-300.

2 (page 29)
Russell, M. A. H. (1990) *op. cit.*

3 (page 29)
Miller, W. R. & Rollnick, S. (1992) *Motivational Interviewing: Preparing people to change.* Guildford Press: New York, London

4 (page 29)
Lewis, C. S. (1942) *The Screwtape Letters*

5 (page 31)
Orleans, C. T. (1985). 'Understanding and promoting smoking cessation'. *Annual Review of Medicine*, 36, 51-61.

6 (page 36)
Tate, J. C. & Stanton, A. L. (1990) 'Assessment of the validity of the Reasons for Smoking Scale'. *Addictive Behaviours*, 15, 129-135.

Chapter 3
7 (page 45)
Cox, B. D., Blaxter, M. & Buckle, A. L. J. (1987) *The Health and Lifestyle Survey.* The Health Promotion Research Trust: London

8 (page 45)

Cohen, S. & Lichtenstein, E. (1990). 'Perceived stress, quitting smoking and smoking relapse'. *Health Psychology*, 9(4), 466–478.

Chapter 4

9 (page 56)

Glantz, S., Barnes, D., Bero, L., Hanauer, P., & Slade, J. (1995). 'Looking through the keyhole at the Tobacco Industry. The Brown and Williamson Documents'. *Journal of the American Medical Association*, 274(3), 219–224.

10 (page 56)

Yeaman, A. *Implications of Batelle Hippo I & II, and the Griffith Filter.* Brown and Williamson Document no. 1802.05. Cited in Glantz et al, 1995.

11 (page 56)

Green, S. (1974). *Notes on the Group Research & Development Conference at Duck Key, Fla.* BW document no. 1125.01, cited in Glantz et al, 1995.

12 (page 56)

Pepples, E. (1976). *Industry response to cigarette health controversy.* (BW Document no. 2205.01.)

13 (page 58)

Russell, M. A. H. (1990) *op. cit.*

Further Support

UNITED KINGDOM
Websites
• NHS website on smoking: **http://www.uglysmoking.info/**
This is an excellent interactive website for smokers who are keen to quit. Packed full of information on the effects of smoking, benefits of quitting, and details of further free smoking cessation support in your area. This website is easy to read and use.

• QUIT – a charity that helps people give up smoking:
http://www.quit.org.uk/
This is an easy-to-use interactive website for people wanting help with quitting. Offers individual advice via e-mail and a telephone help line (see below).

• ASH – Action on Smoking and Health:
http://www.ash.org.uk/
ASH is a campaigning public health charity working to eliminate the harm caused by tobacco. The ASH website contains information on a whole range of smoking-related issues, from fact sheets about nicotine addiction, effects of smoking, benefits of quitting and tips to help you quit, to tobacco control legislation, recent news about their campaigns and so on. There are many links to other sites including quitting smoking sites. ASH is evidence-based and cites a lot of research which makes some of the information quite technical and not particularly easy to read.

Telephone support
These are free, confidential telephone services for all smokers. Trained advisers can provide you with information, advice and support about

quitting and referrals to local programmes and services in your community.

- **NHS Smoking Help-line: 0800 169 0 169**
- **QUIT Help-line: 0800 00 22 00**

AUSTRALIA
Websites
- Quit Now – The National Tobacco Campaign
http://www.quitnow.info.au/index2.html
The website of the Australian National Tobacco Campaign. The site is a one-stop-shop including a Quitters' page, online advice and a free quit pack. A user-friendly, interactive site which combats smoking through advertisements with graphic images of damage caused by smoking. These images can be powerfully motivating but can also put smokers off. If you feel looking at images will not help, just ignore them and focus on the useful information provided on this site. Includes advice on how to quit in eight different languages.

- ASH – Action on Smoking & Health, Australia
http://www.ashaust.org.au/

NEW ZEALAND
Websites
- The Quit Group
http://www.quit.org.nz/
The Quit Group co-ordinates national smoking cessation programmes to help New Zealanders quit smoking. These services include a quit-line offering free support and advice, and quit cards, a programme that lets health providers with an interest in smoking cessation register to distribute exchange cards for patches or gum to smokers wanting to quit. This is an interactive site for quitters, with information on quitting and links to further support and advice:

• ASH – Action on Smoking and Health in New Zealand
http://www.ash.org.nz/home.php

Telephone Support
• The Quitline: Support from the Quit Group (see above): 0800 778 778

SOUTH AFRICA
Websites
• The Heart Foundation, South Africa
http://www.heartfoundation.co.za/s_nosmoke.
The website of the South African Heart Foundation includes pages on smoking. Provides information on dangers of smoking, and tips to help you quit.

CANADA
Websites
• Canadian Health Network: Health Info For Everyone.
http://www.canadian-health-network.ca/
Contains lots of information on tobacco and smoking, including advice and support for those wanting to quit. Includes many links to other sites.

• Canadian Cancer Society
http://www.cancer.ca/
Includes web pages on cancer prevention by stopping smoking. Offers a detailed step-by-step plan for quitting and telephone support – see below.

Telephone Support
Run by the Canadian Cancer Society:

Manitoba	1 877 513-5333
New Brunswick	1 877 513-5333

Nova Scotia	1 877 513-5333
Ontario	1 877 513-5333
Prince Edward Island	1 888 818-6300
Quebec	1 888 853-6666
Saskatchewan	1 877 513-5333

The Smokers' Helpline is a free, confidential telephone service for all smokers, whether or not they are ready to quit. Trained quit specialists can provide you with information, advice and support, along with print resources and referrals to local programmes and services in your community. They can also assist family and friends who would like to help a smoker quit.

Although the Canadian Cancer Society does not run telephone helplines in the other provinces, it gives the following numbers for helplines run by other organisations:

British Columbia	1 877 455 2233
Alberta	1 866 332 2322
Newfoundland	1 800 363 5864

INTERNATIONAL

All the above websites are, of course, available all over the world. While the information on local resources will be of limited use, the information on the websites is universally applicable and may be useful to everyone.

Index